SHOW UP
for
Yourself

**How to Overcome Postpartum Depression, Lose Weight,
and Keep It Off for Good**

TAE RENÉ

Disclaimer

I'm not a nutritionist, physician, nor fitness trainer. Please consult with a medical expert before adhering to this personal advisory.

Contents

Dedication iv

Introduction v

My Message to You vi

Chapter 1   The Renovation 1

Chapter 2   The Birth of the Emotional Wardrobe 4

Chapter 3   The Birth of Ella 7

Chapter 4   For the Love of Jackie 14

Chapter 5   The Snap UP 18

Chapter 6   The Modern-Day Renaissance Woman 22

Chapter 7   Elevate Your Mentality 25

Chapter 8   The Pursuit of Transformation 33

Chapter 9   Commit to the Climb 43

Chapter 10 The Best Revelation, Ever 56

Chapter 11 Faith Over Fear 63

Chapter 12 Post to Be 69

Chapter 13 Crop Top Conformity 75

Chapter 14 The Postpartum Pandemic 79

Chapter 15 "Black" on Track 83

Chapter 16 Marathon-Minded 86

Chapter 17 Representation Matters 98

Chapter 18 Imperfection to Progression 105

Chapter 19 Why Not, Wellness? 116

Chapter 20 Heirs of Strength 124

Dedication

I would like to dedicate this
book to my beautiful daughters, Ella and Ever.
Thank you for revealing my power.
Mommy loves you.

Introduction

"For my strength is made perfect in weakness."
—II Corinthians 12:9

It is often in times of weakness that we discover our strengths. An unyielding faith-posture led me to persistence in restraint, spiritual ambition, and unforeseen character development. Following an outpour of questions and demands for insight, I've mustered the tenacity to unveil the narrative of my transformational postpartum weight loss journey.

I am Tae René. I'd considered myself a strong woman until my hope was invaded by an unexpected weakness. During a time that society deems to be the happiest period of a woman's life, I was overwhelmed with fear.

It is here that I will convey what I had to lose to win in each consequent battle. Truthfully, the compromise was fundamental for the evolution of my womanhood. With the weight of postpartum depression looming, I lost 130 pounds. I lost 61 pounds the first time and 69 pounds subsequently.

Reaching your ideal weight begins when the search for the "perfect" diet ends. I am going to introduce you to my life and how I showed up daily for my family, celebrity clients, and, most importantly, myself. I was able to drop the weight physically and mentally. So buckle up as we embark on a journey to self-assurance, an endless awareness, and confidence beyond measure.

My Message to You

I would like to preface this book by informing you that you are beautiful exactly the way you are. You know why? Fortunately, you are the byproduct of your story, and you won! Gratitude is the gateway to greatness. Recognize that you are a survivor; you are beautiful and can go exceedingly further.

This book is for women, especially mothers who want to transform their lives physically, spiritually, and mentally to rediscover their power and beat the inevitable life-balancing acts of motherhood, career, love, and self. Each day you show up for your children, you show up for your companions, you show up for your career, and now it's time for you to show up for yourself.

There is a multitude of women who struggle to initiate their wellness journey. You are not alone. The biggest misconception about weight loss is that it is only a physical endeavor. Beneath those complex layers of skin lies an internal guidance awaiting its activation. Generally, most women are unaware of the force of this tool. In this intimate exposition, I hope to ignite one revelation: that you are more than a conqueror and can arrive at the pinnacle of your essence when you win the war within.

"When you don't prioritize showing up for yourself, you get the leftovers of life's daily demands."

TAE RENÉ

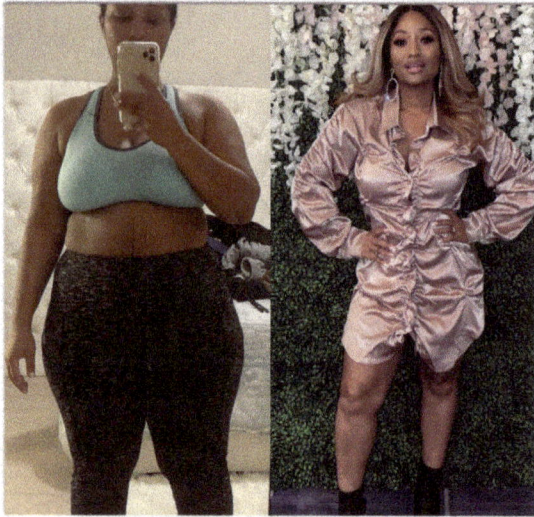

Before & After

1

The Renovation

When you don't prioritize showing up for yourself, you get the leftovers of life's daily demands. This inverted approach prevents you from reaching your fullest potential. Consequently, the energy you have left is dedicated to instant gratification, such as streaming television shows and movies, dining out and drinking with friends, or aimlessly scrolling on social media. But hey, you deserve it after meeting everyone else's demands for the day, right? How many times have you identified with this feeling?

Have you ever heard the next level of your life will demand a different version of you? Well, that is the you that you're showing up for! Have you ever heard the quote, "Make your dreams so big that you have to reinvent yourself to meet them?"

Reinvention is the process through which something is changed so much that it appears entirely new. Let the renovations begin, shall we?

The first matter of change is not the food that you indulge in. That's merely the tip of the iceberg. Delectable foods are masked as freedom, but when unwrapped, it holds you captive in a foreign body struggling between your appearance and self-worth. I want to encourage you to avoid this viscous cycle of having another short-lived orgasmic food experience that distances you from your personal goals.

Through self-reflection and discipline, I recognized the power of my strength to uproot unhealthy eating habits, toxic thoughts, anxiety, and depression. This required a liberal amount of unapologetic honesty and introspection. However, these tools will enable you to show up for yourself and achieve a renewed life of confidence and joy.

"We Roar. Hence We War"

"Fragility was the antithesis of my mother and grandmother's color preference when it came to displays of their emotional wardrobe. I descended from a lineage of strong women. Unlike me, my heart has been practically sown on my sleeve as emotional paraphernalia. My predecessors contradict the fundamental character delicacies encouraged as traditional feminism. Appropriately selfless, gentle, and compliant are all unvoiced expectations— until permitted to lie on our backs in surrender to the unknown when we're entitled to roar and scream at the top of our lungs as a full being extensively stretches through our magical valley of life and birth transpires. We war. Hence, we roar."

TAE RENÉ

2

The Birth of the Emotional Wardrobe

Covered in teenage tears, I ran to the kitchen table where my granny sat at the head. Her throne is how I've always referenced it. No one else would dare mock her honor and seat themselves there.

My glassy eyes gazed upon her, raised eyebrows and tilted head of honey blonde curls as I sat across. "I just don't understand, Granny," I said in pity.

I truly expected a moment of consolation followed by a lengthy speech, but never did I think I could brace myself for what was to come from her mouth.

"Are you weak?"

"Ma'am?" I asked, perplexed.

"Are you weak?"

I said, "No, ma'am," fearing disappointing her, unsure if my tears disqualified me from her honor.

"No one deserves your tears. You understand?" she said with her finger pointed and lips tight, reminiscent of the exact way my mom's would curl when she means what she says, leaving no room to inaccurately discern the gravity of her words.

"Yes, ma'am," I replied with my chin up militantly.

Deep down, I hoped I could deliver on this abrupt initiation. The emotional wardrobe was evident. We were strong women. In contrast, my mother's response to my adolescent boy-frenzy issues was a tad lighter in approach than my granny's, yet, yielded the same results. You see, she would equip me with a little more strategy.

"Did they hurt you?" she asked.

She could hear my shame of silence through the opposite end of our call. "What's the rule, Shonté? Give it three days, and the pain will ease up, but keep your head held high."

Although there were 800 miles wedged between us, as I'd left Flint, MI in 2007 to pursue my dreams in Atlanta, I lived by her words.

In moments of dismay, I learned to borrow an item or two from their emotional wardrobe collection until I acquired a collection of my own. Strangely, I applied this mechanism to my wellness journey. I often clothed myself in this fortitude, especially in the beginning.

"Being broken helps you realize that you're unbreakable."

TAE RENÉ

3

The Birth of Ella

I began my wellness journey as a means of survival. It was a means of escape from a sudden attack of postpartum depression. At 41 weeks, I gave birth to a beautiful, healthy baby girl. I was instantly overcome with fear when the doctor put her in my arms. At 25 years old, my life was a compilation of failed missions, fainted friendships, a mountain of student loan debt, an incomplete degree, and an abundant overcast of uncertainty. My future forecasted nothing but obscurity. I felt like I was living a life that I didn't recognize.

There was so much promise in Ella's eyes. They looked exactly like mine. It was as if I was staring back at myself. It was surreal. I imagined what my life would be like if I had a fresh start, and that's exactly what I wanted to give her. I felt the pressure to make her life everything that mine wasn't. I wanted her to have a stable household and family. I wanted to be perfect in every way.

My heart was constantly tugged between paralyzing fear and awe. We named her after that beautiful woman I once knew, the one with the honey blonde curls that inspired my first emotional wardrobe piece, my grandmother, Ella Mae. Keeping the E and the M, we saw fit to name her Ella Monroe. Mommy's little diva.

As much as I prepared for her physical arrival, nothing could have prepared me for the internal challenges ahead. My capabilities to complete the mission of motherhood wavered from day to day.

My mother was only able to stay with me for four weeks. In the weeks following, I had to show up for Ella in a way that I didn't even know existed! Sleep-deprived and burdened by my perceived misfortune of accolades, there was a darkness that overshadowed my joy in an inarticulable way. The emotional wardrobe I wore for years no longer suited me.

The complexities of my unhappiness were beyond what I could unpack alone—even though I wasn't. My goal went from reaching my life-long dreams to surviving the day with a newborn baby and trying to love myself. I'd lost my sense of purpose and didn't know what it would take to reactivate my power.

Identity trials make you question your value and view the world from a completely different vantage point. Motherhood abruptly shifted my life in a way that I did not anticipate. Nevertheless, despite the conditions, I persisted as most moms do, notwithstanding my deteriorating emotional wellness.

Never in a million years did I envision going from 128 lbs. with unmarked skin to over 180 lbs. with a stretch-marked shapeless figure. I literally couldn't look at my reflection without repulsion. In total, I had gained 61 pounds during this pregnancy. My pre-pregnancy weight was around 128 lbs., and I was 189 lbs. postpartum. My grandmother bore six children, and although it was evident, even in her old age, it was not nearly as bad. I felt like damaged goods and knew that this damage was irrecoverable.

My full expectation was that my body would return exactly how it was. Call me naïve, but I was not privy to the fact that my body was the collateral damage in childbirth. How many postpartum bodies had you witnessed by the age of 25? Well, allow me to speak from my own experience. I saw my mother's and grandmother's bodies as a child, but they had already had children, so I had nothing to measure it against besides my own body.

Six months later, I was 25 years old and could not even look at myself. This was literally the most traumatic physical experience I'd undergone. *My life is over.* I thought. I had no doubt that this body would rob me of my future. "Why me?" I questioned. I had no idea how to navigate my life in this physical condition, and what I could see physically couldn't even compete with the internal depreciation. My self-confidence was fleeting, and I'd experienced an emotional paralysis that left me idle.

I decided to present my concerns to my doctor during my next OB visit.

"So, do you know how much longer it will take for me to get back to my original weight? And these dark marks, will they ever go away?"

"Oh," she replied. "You know, everyone's body is different. They may go away, and they may not go away. It's a genetic matter."

Thinking back to seeing my mother and grandmother's bodies, I thought, *well, I guess it won't be.*

"Great. Ok, and what about this loose skin around my belly button? For the record, I'm not really eating that much, and I still feel like I look pregnant."

"Oh yeah," she replied. "Well, that should be the least of your worries right now, you know? Eventually, you might want to modify your diet and be a little bit more active, and I'm sure you'll see some progress. In the meantime, do you think you're experiencing any difficulty in caring for your child, or do you feel sad?"

I was an uneducated, 25-year-old young, Black, unwedded woman with a very low income and no family within nearly 1000 miles.

"Oh no! I'm fine."

"Are you sure?" she asked, looking at me intensely. "You don't seem to have the same enthusiasm as you had in previous appointments."

I just looked at her trying to discern her genuineness.

She proceeded, "I have a medication that I can prescribe to you if you need help."

Oh, no! Going back to the root of the Black community, any display of vulnerability will weaken your case of being competent in the world, let alone independent. We've been conditioned to believe that even if you feel weak, they should never know. It will only be leveraged against you in the least expected moment. My theory is that this defense mechanism is a result of multigenerational oppression and discrimination. We coped with our emotions the best way we could. As the doctor waited for my reply, I could hear my grandmother saying, "Are you weak?"

I'm not even mad at such a mechanism being instilled in me during my youth. We all have an emotional wardrobe. We safeguard our transparency as a means of protection. We've been accustomed to protecting our image and our dignity for centuries. Hence, therapy has been highly feared in the Black community. We were taught to keep our "business" to ourselves, but what was considered an unspoken gospel decades ago is now a corrupted concept.

This was my moment to express myself, my own feelings, my own truth. However, this was not that redefining moment.

"No, I'm fine," I replied.

Of course, feeling one hair away from emptiness and regret as I departed, I called my unofficial psychologist, my best friend—my mother.

"Mom, why didn't you tell me that my body was going to look like this?" I asked in such grief. "And why didn't you tell me I would have to survive on 1 to 2 hours of sleep? How did you do this?"

She replied, "Huh? What do you mean, baby?"

"Mom, I'm literally waiting for my body to go back to the way that it was, and the doctor just told me that it may never go back."

Her response was, "Well, honey, that's what happens when you have kids."

I was mortified; I felt betrayed! In retrospect, I'm tickled by it.

"I needed preparation for this!" I said jokingly in all seriousness.

I knew that if sadness or depression were even implied in the subtext of this conversation, she would have been on the first flight to Atlanta. Subject change, please!

Since food was my trauma response to adversity, uncertainty, and all things uncomfortable, I ate my heart out after that conversation. My emotional eating habits always got the best of me.

Emotional eating is when you consume food as a means to stabilize your emotions. I developed some very toxic habits. It started in my early 20s. I would moderately binge on unhealthy foods, and when I became overwhelmed with guilt, I would drink a bottle of Magnesium Citrate, thinking that this would reverse the effects of my reckless eating.

When battling a sudden unfathomable amount of darkness, bombarding your family and friends with your problems is typically your last resolve. Being a stay-at-home mom, I had a lot of time on my hands. This time consisted of maternal demands, house chores, and recycled TV entertainment. As time progressed, all my days began to look the same, and the absence of my purpose began to surface. This void became unbearable.

As Black women, we've been taught to carry our burdens to the altar, and then in following, we do what? Wait on the Lord, as instructed by our elders. No results? Then you know the good gospel. "He ain't gone put more on you than you can bear." So here I was, waiting and bearing.

Each morning I would wake up, open my Bible app, and read the scripture of the day. I would watch sermons from Joseph Prince, Joyce Meyer, and Creflo Dollar, awaiting a glimpse of hope as the elders promised. My re-awakening began transpiring little by little. Soon enough, I had the courage to confront the truth. Motherhood is not a one size fits all experience.

Can you imagine being on the receiving end of a conversation with someone exclaiming that they don't have the energy to carry out the visions that once fueled their ambitions? That they're running on E, and they feel that they're pouring from an empty cup? That they're exhausted beyond comprehension, and they just want to escape? Except, that's not an option because there's no time for discovery. They have to be responsible for their children and meet every one of their needs.

Additionally, their body has suffered so much distress that they hate looking at themselves in the mirror, and the thought of being intimate is mortifying. Although they wouldn't actively pursue ending their lives, they wouldn't mind if God didn't wake them the next day. If someone entrusted you with this information, think of how you would respond. This behavior is not exactly recognized as common postpartum behavior.

Each step of the way, I ensured that I put my best foot forward, especially when it came to nursing, which was a foreign concept in my family. The health benefits of nursing far outweighed any discomfort that I was experiencing. Besides, I was also looking forward to the complimentary weight loss.

Breastfeeding was the most magical assignment I've ever seen my body perform. I was in awe that if I saw past the pain, my body could give my children absolutely every single immunity essential. The only requirement was me. I was all she needed. This incomparable connection is something I'd never experienced. This further confirmed that there is no hood like motherhood.

The disclaimer, however, is that you have to eat enough calories to produce enough milk. According to Women's Health Magazine, nursing alone allows you to burn 300-500 calories per day. Surely after nursing for four months, I would be able to reclaim my fine in no time! Not quite. Though I'd committed to breastfeeding for months, I'd only lost 10 lbs. I was devastated. I didn't recognize the person staring back at me when I looked in the mirror.

Depression shouldn't be a one-woman battle after bearing children, but it has been for years in America. The only thing that could have de-escalated my depression was more emotional and physical preparation.

Motherhood hit me like a ton of bricks. Over time, I learned to remove one brick at a time to make the load lighter, and eventually, I was able to come out of that dim hole and see the light again. However, no two postpartum journeys are the same.

Unfortunately, I could not think of an open forum to share my inner struggles at this time of my life. My goal is to continue spreading awareness of postpartum depression in the Black community so we can openly embrace one another and heal together.

"*Love is the Strength that fuels true Sisterhood.*"

TAE RENÉ

4

For the Love of Jackie

I remember being at the receiving end of a conversation with my best friend from childhood. We were 13 years old when we met.

Though her talent was promising, her future became short-sighted after the birth of her second child.

She would call me and say, "I don't know what to do, Tae. I want to get out of here."

I would reply, "Okay, well, let's devise a plan and figure it out."

She was so talented. I envisioned her coming to Atlanta and thriving in cosmetology.

In her low moments, she often ranted about the toxic relationship with her child's father and his family. She had recently given birth to her second child after a 5-year break. Afterwhile, she became unrecognizable to me. Though we were miles apart, I could hear her brokenness in our phone conversations. I later learned after visiting her that she had some unresolved trauma from childhood. She developed epilepsy and was prescribed medication to regulate her condition.

The combination of built-up trauma, stress, toxicity in her relationship, her loss of purpose, the responsibility of motherhood, and lack of support all became too much. One day, she called me, and in knowing that I needed time to sit and listen to talk with her, I didn't answer. I told myself I would call her back.

A week passed when another friend called, and I answered the phone.

"Hey, girl! Shonté, are you okay?" she asked.

I said, "Yeah, why wouldn't I be? What's wrong?"

"I'm sorry. Oh my God."

"What is it?"

She said, "It's Jackie."

"What's going on? What---"

The words couldn't come out of my mouth fast enough before she uttered that Jackie had died. She was 28 years old. I don't think I could breathe because I screamed for so long.

I could have been there for her, but I didn't know how. I didn't know how serious it was. I didn't know what she needed. I didn't recognize it. I couldn't identify it. Then I went through it, and I understood.

Jackie's last epileptic episode took place in her sleep. If I were still around, I don't think her life would have taken the turn it had. Though she was one year younger, she was my protector and always had my back. This was my opportunity to have hers. I felt guilty for not protecting her from life's calamities or at least guiding her through them. She was so full of life. I will always remember her for her beauty, outspokenness, sense of humor, and feistiness. My best friend would have done anything for me.

I carried that guilt and pain for years. I honor her memory by sharing with you and teaching women around the world how to show up for themselves even in their darkest days.

"Never allow someone else's journey to define your success."

TAE RENÉ

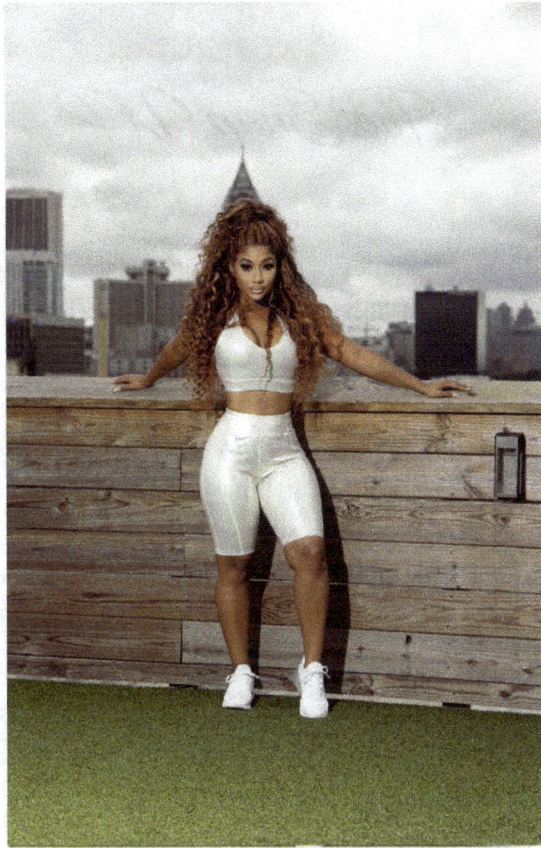

My Snap Up

5

The Snap UP

Do you find yourself aimlessly scrolling on social media, getting lost in a rabbit-hole of content, only to lead you into a depth of wonders, asking yourself why you haven't reached the lifestyle you're witnessing on the screen before you? You, too, may be affected by this disorder.

Hi everybody, my name is LaShonté, and I am recovering from IAD – Internet Addiction Disorder. Okay, I may have exaggerated a little bit, but IAD is a REAL thing!

Of course, we can all be guilty of envying those who "snap back" postpartum. If you are unaware, snap back is an unofficial term that refers to postpartum bodies reverting to their original condition in almost no time. Let me just say that I commend those who are capable of this. However, that word insults those whose bodies don't instantly revert to their pre-baby physiques.

Truth be told, many women that have already undergone cosmetic procedures snap back faster than others. In most cases, once you've had a surgical procedure such as liposuction and have given birth, your body will revert to its prepartum dimensions.

Logging into social media before my eyes are fully opened is a former morning reflex of mine. Social media has become our largest source of entertainment and inspiration. The competition used to be really thin before the evolution of social platforms. I remember when (now I can officially say back in my day) we were in high school. You would hear of another popular person and have no idea what they actually looked like until you met them. Our competition used to be environmental, but now it seems that we're comparing our lives with people we have never even met. We went from being big fish in a little pond to little fish in a big pond.

The pressure is real! Everyone is not who they "pose" to be on social media, or should I say "post" to be. I've been guilty of it myself in the past.

There's so much pressure on women to look a certain way, behave a certain way, take care of our children a certain way, take care of our homes, be married by a certain age, take care of our husbands and families in a certain way, and conduct ourselves in a certain way. Women just have so much pressure on them. And you mean to tell me that we have to heal a certain way? The audacity!

The distress of my body was a major contribution to postpartum depression, in addition to discovering that reaching my long-term goals was too far-fetched to think about and had been reduced to self-sufficiency and survival. I just wanted to take care of my baby, get through the day, and wake up the next day. I felt alone.

I was celibate for one year after having my first child. I was trying to do everything the right way, but it was literally killing me. Sounds horrible, right? But it's my truth. I had to rely on God and His Word that says tomorrow has enough worries of its own and live for the day. I had a daughter to raise and a life to live. I had to rely on His strength. The weight of postpartum depression did not allow me to embrace the future.

Now that I've reached my weight loss goal, people often approach me, saying, "Ooh girl, you snapped back."

I cringe! Every single time. There is such a difference between working to reach your physical goals and reaching them by genetic design.

Now, I take a deep breath and politely reply, "No, I'm sorry this was more of a resurrection than a snapback."

A part of me had to die to make room for the rebirth of my new and improved identity.

So if anything, snapbacks should refer to snapping back into the essence of who you are and how to navigate the world. In fact, let's just cancel the physical snapback culture and embrace a culture that allows women to heal and rediscover the core of who they are. We're only moving forward and upward from here. Our focus should be to snap up and not snapback.

The reality is that when we give birth to our children, we give birth to an unknown version of ourselves. Motherhood is a journey, not a destination. In hindsight, it allowed me to reset and really delve into the soul of my womanhood.

"I can do ALL things through Christ who strengthens me."

PHILIPPIANS 4:13

6

The Modern-Day Renaissance Woman

In the African culture, the phrase "it takes a village to raise a child" is literal.

"Do you have any more help with the baby?" my good friend asked me after my mom returned to Michigan after my daughter's birth.

"No."

"Wow. In my country, when women give birth, a helper called an au pair comes to live with them, cooks meals, and helps care for them and their baby. Your sisters are also responsible for your recovery. They give you massages and herbs and make special foods for you to heal your body."

In contrast, although the United States is one of the most developed countries in the world, it has low regard for postpartum recovery. The 900,000 women who suffer from postpartum depression annually are allotted eight weeks of maternity leave. That speaks to the nature of America's regard for postpartum recovery. There is no wonder that approximately 1 in 10 women experiences postpartum depression.

Did you know that some European countries offer parental leave for six months to a year? It is known that the United States has the least maternity leave available for its citizens.

In addition to nursing our young, we have to compete with male counterparts in our careers, make it home on time to get dinner ready for the family, complete our children's bedtime routine, and get settled for bed with good hygiene and an inviting smile and do it all again the next day with grace.

Mothers are due restitution in America, whether it's an increase in pay, free grocery delivery for the rest of our lives, discounted childcare, a free fitness membership, one spa day per year, or two free lunches out of the year. A notion of some kind that extends beyond a commercialized holiday to make us feel appreciated for taking on such a physical, emotional, and spiritual journey. For goodness' sake, we bring forth life at the expense of our own.

We are no longer who we were before we gave birth, yet we are trying to perform at the same level with this added responsibility. It is impossible to return to the original routine of caring for our homes, careers, relationships, and personal lives. Not to mention, the expected performance rate in all of these roles is 100%. I believe postpartum depression becomes evident in our lives when we do not balance our roles. You must create a new normal that works for you. When in doubt, remember,

"I can do all things through Christ who strengthens me."
—Philippians 4:13

Recently, I had a revelation when I read this scripture, and since I've never looked at it the same. It no longer referred to anything that I wanted to do. It referred to everything that I wanted to do. I want to share this revelation with you. Don't base your potential on your current circumstances. You can be a mother, a boss in your career, have a healthy love life, and look and feel your best because God strengthened you to do it all. How many things can you do through Christ who strengthens you? All things!

"There's no elevator to success.
You have to take the stairs."

ZIG ZIGLAR

7

Elevate Your Mentality

So how do we go from being normal everyday women to these goal-crushing conquerors? Here's what you do:

- You acknowledge each defeating thought that attempts to invade our minds.
- Combat those thoughts by replacing them with thoughts that evoke positive emotions.
- Utilize the art of sound, scent, and sight if we need help activating these feelings within us.

The better you feel, the more likely you will succeed on your wellness path. Your emotions, thoughts, and actions are all connected. Your choices directly result from this formula. **Keep in mind that there is a difference between being the best version of yourself and the best duplicate of another.**

Addiction

I'm reading a book called *Purpose Driven Life* by Rick Warren. In this book, I learned that addictions are not removed but replaced. Generally, addiction is often associated with substance abuse. However, far more relationships can be classified as toxic, and our relationship with food is one of them. In my personal experience, I've learned that if we are going to replace a negative habit, it has to be in exchange for something much greater, something that will fulfill your every need.

Meet your new best friend, ally, and accomplice, the one that complements your promise. You're going to fall in love with her. Her name is purpose. The most influential key to my success was the pursuit of purpose. I recognized during my postpartum journey that the vacancy in my mission was holding me captive.

Being unclear will confine you to a space that is hard to break through unless you have an accurate perception of yourself. Nothing except walking in your purpose will fill that void, the void that you attempt to fill with gluttony, alcohol, sex, overindulgence in social media, and toxic television. It's a vicious subconscious cycle. This common behavior is disguised as contentment, but it's rooted in dream deprivation and denial. I had to surrender my will to God to live a purpose-filled life.

Various religions exercise the importance of faith, and more importantly, they emphasize strength in the act of surrendering. This is the next most instrumental tool in your wellness journey. There are different acts of surrender. We normally resist surrender because of pride and ego. We believe it is a cowardly act, but it is actually a courageous one and your strongest weapon in the pursuit. When you decide to transform your life, you release yourself to reveal the beauty that you possess inside.

To surrender spiritually means to give up your personal will for God's will. This allows you to access and experience God in a way you never have. Insanity is doing the same thing and expecting different results. If you want something you've never had, you have to do something you've never done. Leaving your comfort zone requires a drastic change, and I always seek God first to ensure that I'm in alignment.

"You don't have to see the whole staircase. Just take the first step."
—Martin Luther King

One step, one workout, one pound, one meal, one thought, one day. That is how you navigate on this path to wellness. Don't bombard yourself with thoughts of how uncomfortable this will be. Remember, this is a marathon, not a sprint. Focus on your evolution and remain marathon-minded. There are many benefits outside of the physical results you will obtain through this experience. When you really want something, the simple pursuit of it is gratifying.

I recall scrolling across a music industry icon sharing motivational counsel on social media that was game-changing. "People are so concerned with what they're gaining in the end that they aren't focused on who they are becoming in the process." I couldn't agree more. Think of this as the conquest of the ultimate you. Don't discount your internal transformation by putting too much emphasis on the exterior.

Triathletes train for marathons year-round. It's called conditioning. You must recondition your minds and bodies to endure the challenges ahead of you with the same diligence. Each day that I remained committed to my wellness journey, whether I lost 5 lbs. or 3 lbs., I appreciated that I was becoming a woman of my word, giving my body the best mental and physical treatment it deserves. Furthermore, I knew that I could trust myself.

How much could you bear if you knew that deliverance was on the other side? If you know that a 30-minute commute will help you reach your desired destination, you will invest everything into arriving. The distance between the body of your dreams and your reality is action.

Going the Distance

When you want to travel somewhere and need directions, you research the location and find the address. You enter the location in your GPS, fill up your gas tank, and go the distance. Time is taken out of the day for the commute and planned accordingly. All factors, such as traffic, detours, gas stations, and even restaurants along the route, are considered. Let's put this into the perspective of weight loss, shall we?

What you want, in essence, would be your destination. You know how to get there, right? Let's consider this your route to reach your desired destination. You have a vehicle, and if you don't, you know someone that does. If that is not an option, then public transportation can be used as a means of transport.

Finally, you need to prepare for this trip. Find the nearest gas station and fuel the vehicle with the appropriate gas grade in order to continue your journey. Thus, reaching our destination is a simple matter of two things: reaching a decision and going the distance.

Weight loss is psychological territory. Do not allow external variables to prevent you from success. Remember, you are the decision-maker; hence, your position is self-imposed. This is nothing like applying for a job promotion. You are not at the mercy of someone else's approval. There is no risk involved. The results are inevitable. You are in control of the way you show up for yourself.

The objective is to always choose long-term success over short-term satisfaction. Once you master this mind-play, the possibilities are endless for you, not just because you will look and feel better but because you've built character through the process that will last a lifetime. The transformation ignited within you sparks fire in your relationships, finances, and career. You know why? Simply because you have chosen to implement the psychological and spiritual principles to claim power over every area of your life.

To assist you in your journey, take a moment to create affirmations to reinforce your decision. An affirmation is a statement written in the present tense that describes you in the future. I want you to write the top three reasons that inspire you to reach your self-care goal. My personal affirmation during my process was, "Living my dreams outweighs my desire for food." It was just that simple. My hunger for change outweighed my dependency on food. As Benjamin Franklin once said, I've learned to *"Eat to live, don't live to eat."*

ASSIGNMENT

1. Write three affirmations, quotes, or mantras in the present tense.

_____

_____

_____

_____

_____

_____

_____

_____

_____

2. Create an album in your photo gallery on your mobile device and name it "Show Up For Yourself." Add a present photo of yourself to this album and name it "Before" with today's date. Leave space for your after photo.

"And do not be conformed
to this world but be
transformed and progressively
changed by the renewing
of your mind."

ROMANS 12:2

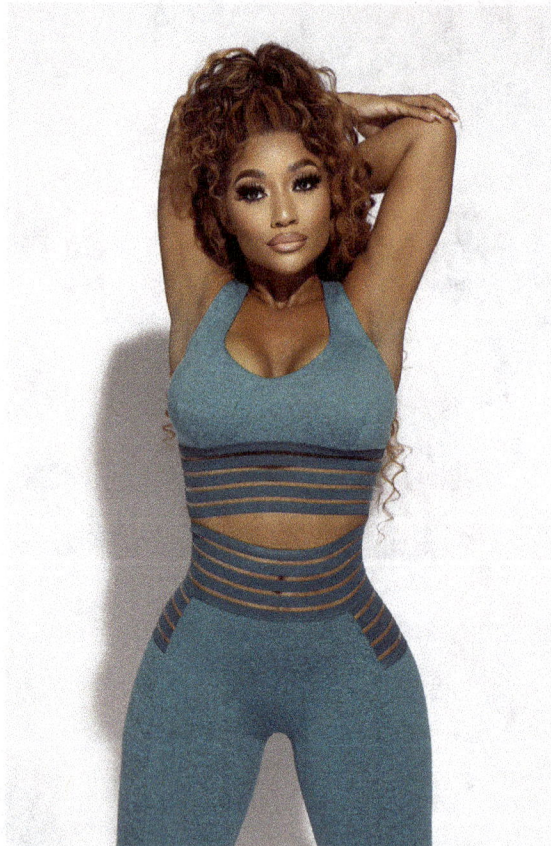

My Pursuit

8

The Pursuit of Transformation

When I began putting more effort into my wellness journey, new business opportunities and relationships emerged. The best investment I've made to date was in restoring my health. It's not a coincidence that things began to unfold as they should when I took action. In the Word of God, it says that faith without works is dead (James 2:20).

I was looking forward to the physical results of my wellness initiative, but this was also a spiritual journey for me. I read my Bible daily, watched a lot of sermons, and listened to many inspirational podcasts. I kept my mind focused on all things positive. I reduced my exposure to toxic music and television. Be mindful of the content you consume. Content gets embedded into our subconscious minds, and we become defeated before getting in the ring to show up for ourselves.

What Do You Want?

We pursue high-paying jobs, nice cars, designer shoes, exotic travel adventures, and the companion of your dreams, for what? Is it for confidence, respect, security, freedom, the laurels of our labor? Is it for more than just "flexing on the 'Gram?" It's for something that has to do with personal gain in some way or another. What you want is relative to who you are and what you want to achieve.

Your definition of a successful and healthy marriage and thriving career may vary from mine; it's all personal, and body goals are no different. I don't believe that there is "the" perfect body. I believe that there is the perfect body for you. I measured my body goals against the body that I once knew. It wasn't a model on the cover of *Vogue Magazine*. I've never had a lean physique; I just wanted to be the best version of myself, and that is what I want for you. I want you to reach your highest potential and go that extra mile for excellence.

This sometimes meant going to the gym every free opportunity I had. It meant going to parties often and not drinking alcohol. It meant showing up for the better version of myself that was awaiting me despite the cost or inconvenience. When you know that you know that you know, all you have to do is the work, and the results will show up.

We see this approach in various aspects of life. Consider a college student pursuing a degree. They do not take all their courses at one time. However, it is one class, one test, one grade at a time. It is beyond a shadow of a doubt that if the college student commits to completing each assignment, they get closer to the goal daily. Similarly, your wellness journey is one meal at a time, one day at a time, one pound at a time to eventually reach your goal size. There is an unequivocal amount of promise in your pursuit.

While I'm using the pursuit of an undergraduate degree as an analogy, I never graduated college. I've attempted to complete my degree three times. Here's when you have to know recognizing your purpose comes into play.

You see, I'm a results-oriented person, and if you present me with the results that I want, I'm going to do whatever it takes to achieve them. That objective was not graduation for me. I know you're probably wondering, "Well, if you had the discipline to lose over 60 lbs. twice, why didn't you have the discipline to complete your degree?"

First and foremost, I am 28 credits away from graduating. I'm so close. Why won't I just push through? A degree is not exactly a prerequisite for what I want to acquire in life. However, relationships, hustle, and experience were essential. This goes hand in hand with your weight loss journey. You have to really want it to commit! If you don't visualize it, you won't see yourself there and work for it! It's plain and simple!

People ask me all the time what I did to lose 70 lbs. *What did you eat? How did you stay consistent? Was it hard?* My answer is initially, "Yes!!" I'm going to be honest with you. The first three days are the worst! However, I persisted because I knew what I wanted! To increase your chances of success, I recommend conducting a self-assessment along your journey. As time progresses, you'll realize what works for you and what doesn't work for you. Each day you collect that data and apply it towards improving day by day.

I changed my undergraduate major three times, which I thought would help me subdue the struggle to be passionate about my educational endeavors since I know that I'm a results-driven person. But there was no reward in suppressing my true dreams for the career expectations of others. I dropped out of college and went directly for what I wanted! I'm not saying I recommend this for everyone. My point is that victory is inevitable when you discover what's worth working for.

Show Up for Your Passion

After the birth of Ella, I fell in love with my talent. After a 4-year hiatus, I picked up my makeup brushes again. Although I didn't know where it would take me, I knew it was something I enjoyed. I knew that beauty had no bounds when it came to makeup. At the time, I discovered some YouTube channels that caught my interest and decided to create one of my own. I had no idea what I was doing. My production consisted of a shade-less lamp, a sleeping baby, and very few tools.

This is why I emphasize the importance of purpose. There is power in the pursuit of purpose. As you are on your purpose-filled journey, you are less consumed with the thoughts and frustrations of hunger. The fulfillment you gain when pursuing your passion outweighs your craving for an unhealthy lifestyle.

Now, of course, lifestyle factors must be considered. Many may argue, "Well, I have a family, and I have to cook for my kids. I'm not cooking two separate meals." Yes, I know, and guess what? You all can eat healthy as a unit. Don't think your way out of this. Remember that this is a lifestyle change and that there is a healthy alternative for every excuse you can think of.

"My hair is natural. I don't have time. I don't know what to do." We make time for the things that we want. Get a wig! I don't care if it's from the beauty supply store or custom-made. Honey, it changed my life. I'm just advocating for the lazy ones like myself that won't jeopardize hair styling because of working out. Sometimes you have to get creative and prioritize. It has resulted in consistency in my workout regimen.

What You're Eating Or What's Eating You?

It's not as much about what you eat as it is about what's eating you. What's causing you to eat things that don't benefit you? What is it that's causing you to continue to consume food that implodes upon your self-confidence? This book is so much bigger than nutritional facts, workouts, and diet plans. This is about changing YOU, and as a result, your habits will follow. It's a natural give-and-take dynamic.

Give-and-take relationships are defined by an exchange of motivated efforts. In this experience, you will give your body something to motivate your mind and vice versa. When we master this psychological exchange, we can tailor our physiological results.

If you don't feel that you're that strong mentally, take the initiative to make the best choice, and your body will follow suit. That's right, even if it's not satisfying now, make the decision! Believe it or not, giving your body what it needs versus what you want conditions you to make better choices in the future. The more conscious I was of what I ate, the less I craved unhealthy foods.

This advisory is being given by someone who grew up with a 5-star southern cooking grandmother. So trust and believe I know how great food can be. My grandmother was from Vidalia, GA; hence, I grew up eating pork chops smothered with gravy over creamy grits with eggs scrambled to perfection. Homemade biscuits, ham, black-eyed peas, cornbread, greens, and neckbones. Let's not even talk about her peppered steak and rice or that homemade pound cake. Sunday dinner at Granny's was the best! Ok, I digress. I am definitely not trying to tempt anyone!

Alternatives to these meals do exist, but nothing compares. Thank the Lord for moderation. You don't have to eliminate everything from your diet in one day; it can be gradual. It took me 15 months after each pregnancy to reach my weight goals, but the second time was the absolute hardest!

I've tried everything you can think of: colonics, calorie counting, keto (no white foods), juicing, raw vegan, lemonade, pescatarian, blood type, plant-based, intermittent fasting, and unfortunately, starvation, which I do not recommend. We're talking about over 11 years of ups and downs! So the question that everyone wants to know is what actually worked.

Different diets worked at different times for different purposes in my life. One thing I've never tried, however, is diet pills. I know that some pills actually work. However, I'm very apprehensive about dietary supplements because I don't want my body to become dependent on substances to burn fat, boost my metabolism, or suppress my appetite.

When considering a new dietary approach, Here's my question: Are you looking for a long-term or short-term solution? All of them worked to an extent. When I wanted quick results and a scalable goal, juicing and calorie counting worked. However, there were times when I would see significant weight loss, only for it to resurface more aggressively.

When I wanted to fit in a dress by Friday, and it was Monday, I would do intermittent fasting combined with what I like to call carb-curving. This is the elimination of carbs in your diet. The weight would disappear but, unfortunately, reemerge as soon as I started back eating anything of substance. Here's the key! There are no shortcuts, beloved! At least none that will provide you with long-term results. Hence, it's critical to conform your life to the success you desire. It's a lifestyle pursuit of showing up for yourself.

Face the Truth

I know what you want to hear, and I can tell you exactly that, but it won't be the truth. The truth is that you know how to lose weight. Yes, I said it. If you don't know how to lose weight, you surely know what causes you to gain it. Yet, the dietary changes you've attempted don't last past your nail appointment. Can we go there? Let us! I'm not making you aware of anything that I didn't confess myself!

It doesn't take a nutritionist to tell us; we know whether the food we put in our mouths will do more harm to our body than good. If a cheeseburger and fries or a grilled salmon salad were entrée options on a menu, which option would be better? The salmon salad, right? Certainly, we know what is best for our bodies.

We are so intentional about how we wear our makeup, how we wear our hair, and who we date because these things are an extension of who we are. We can even go as far as to say they are representations of us. Comparably, the food we ingest has the biggest physical influence, yet we are unintentional about what we eat. The food we consume is also a reflection of us. Or is it? It is evident that you are what you eat. Moreover, you eat what you ARE. Therefore, if you want to change what you produce, you must change what you consume.

Currently, you are living in the physical manifestation of your life's choices. When you wake up in the morning, you decide everything from your toothpaste to your wardrobe. Have you ever gone shopping and deliberately chosen an outfit that doesn't complement you? So, why choose to eat something that doesn't flatter your body or contribute to your physical standards?

If there are some things that you aren't satisfied with, then it's time to pivot your course. The beauty in all of this is that you are the navigator in this great journey of wellness. You are behind the wheel. Once you recognize that your life is a culmination of your choices, you, as the HPICs (Head Pilots In Charge), can easily take a flight to your destination of choice. *You are only one decision away from changing the rest of your life. Don't miss that opportunity!*

Diet plans and fitness videos are one Google search away. Thanks to technology, resources are at our fingertips. If you Google "how to lose weight," I'm confident there will be an overabundance of fitness routines and diet plans. I'm sure all of us have taken this initiative before, but why didn't we apply it? We must pose this question before we move any further.

The most fundamental phase of our work is uncovering why we pursue something that further distances us from who we want to be. Each day, we have an opportunity to do something that our future selves will thank us for. Your former self is thanking you today for taking action. Here's the key: *You MUST first change your MIND.*

Before you lose weight, you must change your mind. It's vital to your consistency. The internal pivot that transpires during your reawakening is one of the most monumental moments of your journey! This mental shift is match-striking! It's revelational! It is groundbreaking, and best of all, it's accessible to you. Let's emphasize your awareness and put less focus on your physical faults.

Take your fears, for example, your dispositions, IQ, thoughts, stimulation, the conception of an idea, or the conception of a child. What do all these things have in common? They are all the source of a product.

Though the process is not always visible, the results are undeniable. Their origin is often overlooked. Your physical transformation is no different.

Unrecognized thoughts produce eating habits, mental endurance, and more. No one can see the change you make inwardly until it manifests physically. Though the depth of this topic is endless, it's safe to say that our psychological transformation is bigger than our physical transformation.

It's time to get in the ring, ladies and gentlemen! Any time boxers get in the ring, they already know everything that there is to know about their competition. This opponent examination process is common for all sports: baseball, basketball, football, soccer, tennis. You name it. When adopting a new wellness strategy, this method is guaranteed to ensure your success. Let's take a look in the mirror and examine your opponent, shall we?

Your biggest competition is you. I'm not talking about the you that wants change. I'm talking about the version of you that will repeatedly show up during this process and tempt you into returning to your former way of thinking, causing you to stumble while climbing to greatness.

Let's use the great character metric of honesty and begin surveying your weaknesses. Your competition (speaking of your soon-to-be former self) is not patient, complains, makes excuses, procrastinates, is unorganized, and is in denial about the possibility of succeeding in this process. The biggest leverage you have is knowing your vulnerabilities so that we can nurture your strengths. Your strength is your awareness. Your awareness aligned you with this book, and it will be instrumental in your conquest.

Here are the strengths to focus on to defeat deficiencies. Exercise the discipline of organization, discipline, intentionality, thought culture, and faith.

ASSIGNMENT

Within the next 24 hours, here's what I want you to do:

When you get out of the shower before you get dressed, I want you to look at yourself in the mirror and ask yourself.

What do you like the most about your body and why?

What areas of your body do you want to improve? Why?

When you reach your body goals, what's the first thing you want to wear?

Now look in the mirror at your opponent and recite this affirmation:

I am beautiful. I am a reflection of God and am determined from this point forward to show up for myself because I need me.

Repeat this to yourself.

My body is a product of my former thoughts and decisions. It is a testament to resilience. From this moment forward, it will be evident that I am well because the choices that I am making align with who I am becoming. I am taking back my power by being intentional about my choices.

I am more than a conqueror.

I am beautifully crafted.

I have authority and power because I'm made in God's image and likeness.

"She is clothed in strength and dignity and laughs without fear of the future."

PROVERBS 31:25

9

Commit to the Climb

Stair climbing is not my favorite exercise, but cardio was one major contributing factor to the success of my wellness journey! I'm not an athlete by any means. I ran track in high school to get in shape for cheerleading, and that was it. I was introduced to running in 2010. I enjoyed how liberated I felt after the completion of each trail. It allowed me time to reflect and be in my own little world. Initially, I could only run across the street before I was out of breath, all jokes aside. I would push myself a few steps further during each run, then 5 minutes of non-stop running became 10, 10 to 15, and before you know it, I was running miles.

Cardio, coupled with what I like to call carb-curving, was undeniably the ultimate key success. I mean, the results were unreal! I topped my regimen off with intermittent fasting, and the game changed. However, my former method didn't work exclusively when I reattempted after birthing my second daughter. Hence, I had to take another approach

Intermittent fasting is one of today's popular health trends. It's defined as a rotational eating pattern. There are various approaches to intermittent fasting, but the only one that I have entertained is the 16:8 intermittent fasting method. The 16:8 intermittent fasting method consists of eating within an 8-hour window and fasting for 16 hours. During that time, it's best to eat protein, whole grains, fruits, nuts, and vegetables.

There are many additional benefits to intermittent fasting. Not only does it supercharge the metabolic rate, which is ideal for sourcing nutrients and calorie consumption in the human body, but it has also been linked to life extension.

When I used this strategy, the weight fell off! Sometimes I would exercise on the elliptical, but most of my fitness routine consisted of running on the treadmill. My workout routine consisted of 30 minutes of cardio at least four times per week. When my eldest daughter, Ella, was younger, working out in the evenings would work best for me. I felt safer running indoors post-dawn. Georgia's weather was too inconsistent to run year-round, so I made the best of running on the treadmill.

I didn't know exactly what I was doing when I worked out. I just knew that it would help me, so I showed up there and did the work. I became more intentional when I realized that doing the work was working. Hence, I began using a fitness app to count my calories. In science, every 3,500 caloric deficit creates one pound of weight loss. Remember when I told you I reenrolled in school about three times? Well, here is a moment when what I learned was actually impactful. During the last half of my pregnancy, I was in school because I didn't know what else to do. That's what you do when you're about to have a child and you're lost and confused. You go to school and go to church! You drive the speed limit, wear your seatbelt, and don't speak unless you're spoken to. Your only friends are TV and Jesus.

One of my courses was kinaesthesis, the study of the body. I resolved that the least I could do was take a course on something I wanted to learn. The science of fitness and weight loss was obviously the best choice. Even if it only provided a glimpse of insight, I figured that I could store it in a mental Rolodex for reference when I needed it.

With this knowledge, I entered all of my stats and personal information; it asked for your current and goal weight. At the time, my weight was 163 pounds, with a goal of 125 pounds. If you decide to use an app it is imperative to log your food each day, it seems redundant and time-consuming, but it was very much worth it. Based on the weight you enter, the app will tell you how many calories you should consume each day and how many weeks it should take to reach your goal. You can also log your workouts.

When I realized that after I consumed about 900 calories and then went running for 30 minutes, it would literally subtract 300 calories, it was game time! I figured out a formula and became consistent with it each day. It became a habit.-I would look forward to logging in to the app, seeing my milestones celebrated, and seeing how much closer I was to reaching my weight loss goal.

You might be wondering, *okay, this is all great, but how did you know what to do at all?* That is a very great point. The first time I executed a successful weight loss strategy was in 2009. I was 20 years old. This is after my relocation from Michigan to Atlanta.

I attended the notorious Michigan State University! Yes, GO GREEN! Let me tell you something about MSU. I lived on the Brody campus. There was a restaurant nearby called Lafayette Square. They used to make custom pasta dishes right before you. First, you would choose your noodles. Secondly, choose a sauce. I always got Alfredo, followed by an assortment of veggies, cheeses, and spices.

I love Italian food, like many Black people. We all know how to whip up some good spaghetti and lasagna, and don't even get me started on pizza.

Lastly, you would top off the meal with a perfectly baked chocolate chip cookie for dessert, which was always fresh. Sometimes I would help myself to two! "I had my way," as my mom and pops like to say. That means you eat until you are satisfied. How could such food be accessible on campus? This felt like 5-star dining! I would eat at Lafayette Square nearly every day, and before I knew it, the pounds were packing on.

College is typically a discovery experience. You're expected to gain 15 pounds during your freshman year since you're taken out of your environment, staying up and studying late. It's where we learn who we are, how we're wired, and what we're willing to work for. During my freshman year,

I gained 20 pounds. I went from 115 pounds to 135 pounds. I lost that full 20 lbs. in 3 months using a similar strategy.

Based on my research and trial and error, I removed all starch from my diet. I was new to the South, so I had to have my sweet tea occasionally. I then began to go to the gym and use the elliptical for at least 30 minutes four times a week. Before I knew it, I went from a size 9 to a size 3.

In hindsight, this is typically the basis of my weight loss approach; however, my next weight loss encounter was more nutritionally sound. It is so bizarre. It seems like it takes 10 minutes or less to gain weight, but it takes 10 days to months to lose. The solution is simple. Replace your desire for short-term satisfaction with long-term desires. As a result of my successful wellness journey in 2009, this became the foundation for my process. It has not ever failed me.

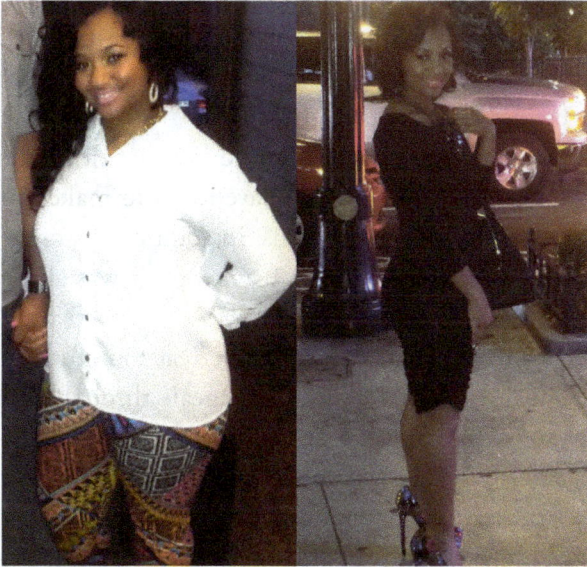

2014
Before & After

Tips for Success

Before attempting this, I recommend a renewed mental approach. Here's what I'd do:

Change your environment: I wore fragrances that made me feel beautiful, listened to uplifting music, gave my attention to inspiring shows, and read new books that enlightened me on my wellness journey.

Pantry Control: Be sure to remove all food from your home that is poor in nutrition and replace them with healthier snacks, such as vegetables, fruit, nuts, and granola.

Keep it tight: Sometimes, I wore clothes that fit kind of snuggly to remind myself that I didn't have room to make the same counterproductive health decisions. In addition, I wore a waist shaper which helped me control my appetite. It was almost impossible to overeat.

Portion control: Make sure you don't eat too much in one sitting. It's much better to spread your meals throughout the day. You should have at least three meals and two snacks in between. That is considered eating five times per day, which signals that your body doesn't need to hold on to the food you ate at previous sittings.

This will increase your metabolism, helping you burn fat faster. Small amounts of nutrients will be released, and little by little, your body will get the nutrition that it needs. Did you know that if you go for extended periods without eating food, your body will store the food for survival?

Stay full: If you drink more water, you will stay full longer. Don't wait until you're hungry to eat. Snack throughout the day and hydrate, hydrate, hydrate! This is a major key! I would sometimes eat even though I wasn't hungry because it kept me from overeating. Keep healthy snacks in your car (nuts, protein bars, and fruit).

Drinking water was one of my biggest challenges and still is to this day. My technique for meeting my water intake goals is to drink it every time I think about it. Start as soon as you wake, and never just sip. Always down a full 16.9 oz bottle or glass of water, whether you're thirsty or not.

Think about it differently: Think of eating as less of an activity and more of a survival function. Find a real hobby and focus on your goals! That's what I'm doing right now by writing this book!

Here's the generic list of healthy foods that you should keep in your home:

Carbohydrates

- Oats
- Potatoes (Sweet/Red Potatoes)
- Bread (Whole-Grain/Whole Wheat/High Fiber Bread)
- Pasta (Whole Grain, Veggie, High Protein, or Fiber)
- Rice (Brown/Jasmine)
- Quinoa

Fats

- Nuts
- Nut Butters
- Avocado
- Olive Oil
- Coconut Oil

Proteins

- Chicken Breast
- Turkey
- Eggs/Egg Whites
- Black Beans
- Legumes
- Chick Peas

- Garbanzo Beans
- Greek Yogurt
- Salmon
- Cod
- Tilapia
- Tuna
- Protein Bars
- Protein Shakes

Vegetables

- Broccoli
- Spinach
- Green Beans
- Cauliflower
- Lettuce
- Carrots
- Collard Greens
- Peas
- Kale

Snacks

- Trail Mix
- Ezekiel Bread with nut butter or fruit spread
- Granola
- Oatmeal or Whole-Grain cereal
- Protein Shakes or Fruit Smoothies

Be mindful of how you incorporate these foods into your diet regimen. If you decide to eat oatmeal for breakfast, whole-grain pasta with sweet potatoes and corn followed by a yogurt parfait for dessert, and have protein shakes in between, you will probably gain weight because your sugar intake would be excessive. Good weight but still weight. Here is where the importance of knowing your macronutrients come into play! The calorie counting app will calculate all of this for you! This is how your caloric intake is determined.

In layman's terms, macronutrients are essentially what the food you consume is composed of. Macronutrient categories are fats, protein, and carbohydrates. Carbohydrates are starches such as potatoes, grains, and sugar. People avoid simple carbohydrates because they are all broken down in the body as one thing, glucose. Complex carbohydrates contain more nutrients and are higher in sugar and fiber. We like fiber because fiber keeps our digestion regulated.

Proteins are something much more complex. Protein is a complex high molecular weight organic compound composed of a long chain of amino acids.

Although many people think that protein is mainly found in meat, broccoli contains more protein per calorie than beef. Also, the protein found in spinach is comparable to fish and chicken. Other sources of protein include potatoes, asparagus, sweet potatoes, mushrooms, brussels sprouts, beans, nuts and more.

Carbohydrates are a macronutrient with which we have a love-hate relationship because aside from fat, we credit carbs as the next main contributor to weight gain. Not to mention almost everyone's weakness contains carbohydrates. We're talking about French fries, pasta, bread, cakes, desserts, almost everything seemingly delightful. Cauliflower is a great substitute for potatoes and rice.

Fiber, sugar and starches are considered carbs. There are whole carbs and refined carbs. I'm sure you've heard people reference a particular food item as processed sugar. Whole carbs, also referred to as complex carbs, include vegetables, quinoa, legumes, potatoes, barley, whole grains, and oats. Refined carbs are unnaturally sweetened drinks and essentially anything made of white flour and white sugar.

Avoid refined sugars because they are digested much quicker than unrefined sugars. They also cause your blood sugar and pressure to spike and can cause instability in your metabolism. Metabolism is defined as the process by which your body converts food to energy.

I needed all the energy I could get to change my life. When incorporating this into my routine, I would be very aware of my macronutrient intake. If not, reality will set in around your waistline as it did mine.

Reality Sets In

I vividly remember my first-time shopping to go out with my girlfriend one night postpartum. This was my first attempt to get cute and meet my girl-friends for cocktails. I went to my neighborhood mall like I would usually, and you know that Forever 21 was popping back then, much like the Zara of today. I said to myself, "Okay, I'm going to go in here and find some black tights and a cute top." I figured tights would conceal my "mommy pooch" the best, and I would still look good if I wore an oversized top.

I searched above and beyond in the store. I didn't find anything that caught my eye. I found a hot pink dress that I liked and a blue dress with a little ruching. A girl loved ruching back then because the gathered fabric concealed my rolls and cellulite very well. I said to myself in confidence, "Okay, I may be able to make this work."

I went into the dressing room and undressed. Looking at my reflection at this time was beyond challenging. I felt sorry for myself. Eventually, I got up the courage to slip on the dress. It didn't come past my thighs. It was a size extra-large. When I asked the store associate if they had a larger size, she said, "No, I'm sorry." This was before the plus-size fashion evolution. I didn't even try on the other dress. I felt so defeated and internally humiliated. I grabbed a blouse and some tights and checked out as soon as possible. One thing about postpartum depression is that it magnifies your shortcomings.

The issue is that I may have been a little full of myself prepartum.

There were some things that I wasn't satisfied with about my body, but I felt that I could run with the best. I didn't have much action in the back and wasn't necessarily racked up top. However, heads turned when I put effort into my look.

There was an imperceptible battle between the version of me that I once knew and the new version of me. I knew that the former version of myself would look at this girl and feel relieved that she was not me. She may have said a prayer for her along the way and befriended her, but she would surely be thankful that she was not in her shoes.

This is how I saw myself postpartum. Except there was no walking away from this girl. I was the girl. In retrospect, it was one of the most humbling experiences I'd ever gone through. The world didn't treat me differently; it was me. I questioned my value each time I glanced at myself, knowing I wasn't giving my best. Although I wanted the LaShonté back that could dance confidently in a crop top and low-rise jeans, I prayed to God that He would bless me to look normal—simply recognizable.

"The Breakthrough is in you"

PASTOR TOURÉ ROBERTS

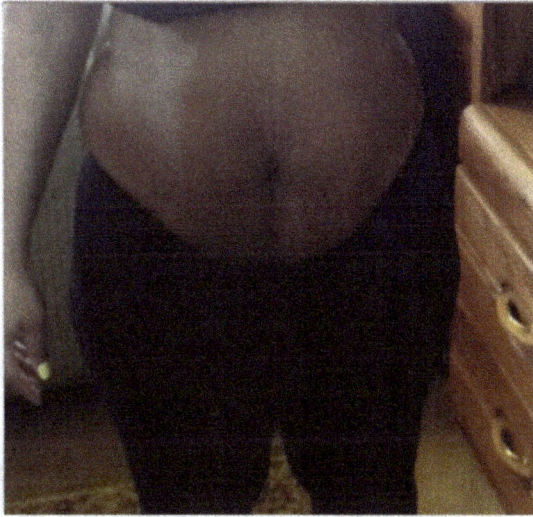

My Tummy

10

The Best Revelation, Ever

I'm always listening for God's voice. Early one morning, while en route to service a client, I sought God for wisdom. I am an avid audience member of "One," a podcast led by Pastors Touré Roberts & Sarah Jakes Roberts.

This particular morning, Pastor Touré was speaking on the subject of breakthroughs. I just remember him repeatedly saying, "The breakthrough is in you! The breakthrough is in you!"

Could my prayers have been answered? I had been praying for confirmation from God because I've been awaiting a breakthrough in my finances and career. I wasn't in a bad position but wanted more for myself. I aspired for prosperity and career elevation. While listening, my perspective shifted, but I didn't understand it quite as well as I do now.

In the recent discovery of my second pregnancy, I was unclear about my future direction. I had recently become engaged, and my fiancé and I were in the process of establishing a foundation. We were house hunting, paying off debt, and doing all of the ideal adult planning. In our minds, it was not the most convenient time to family plan.

I thought to myself, *God, how is a breakthrough in me? Are you referring to this baby? Is this baby going to be the black Bill Gates or Serena Williams?* It didn't make sense until this very moment. I now understand that 3:11 p.m. on July 16, 2021, was a prophecy.

God revealed to me that the breakthrough was the transformation I'm experiencing right now. This revelation resulted from the fast I committed to on June 8, 2021. It's come full circle.

When I encounter times in my life where I feel that I can't hear God's voice, I fast. This removes all distractions and all outside noise.

My second postpartum experience was a breakdown that only God could see me through. I gave birth to my beautiful baby girl on December 10, 2019. I was grieving but prepared for whatever challenges were before me. Despite it all, I knew I had to do something very similar to the survival of my first experience.

One night, when everyone was asleep, I knelt beside my bed and surrendered my will to God. There were so many reasons behind this. I felt like whatever I was pursuing no longer fulfilled me. We all know what that can lead to, a downward spiral of overindulgence and resentment.

The outbreak of the pandemic changed my postpartum experience tremendously. If there was a time that you were ever certain about anything, the imaginary rug of safety was snatched from under just about everyone amid the onset of the Coronavirus. The remains of my career and my improved financial position kept me a little more hopeful than my previous postpartum experience. I was in the discovery process of my purpose the first time around. This time I was somewhat more established. I had a secure clientele, and my husband was doing fairly well in his career.

Yet, my mood shifts began to extend beyond my own personal reach. When the walls began to close in on me, my hope remained. I wasn't going to allow myself to reach the point of defeat I felt during my first pregnancy, which almost evoked an emotional paralysis of my ambition. But these girls! These beautiful, bright-eyed babies gave me hope. They needed me, and they needed me healthy and whole.

My girls were my biggest motivation in my postpartum recovery. I did whatever was necessary to give them the proper love and care they deserved. Although I was entering a foreign territory trying to manage a home, being married and now having two children and working, I was determined to make it work with or without the ideal family support.

I can't believe I'm experiencing this insightful moment as I write. In my efforts to impart knowledge of wellness, I've reached the biggest enlightenment of my entire life. I'm so grateful to have been restored BEYOND my own strength through GOD'S POWER.

The breakthrough Pastor Touré was referring to was my most recent physical, spiritual, and mental transformation. This transformation would not have occurred if I didn't encounter the second postpartum experience with my baby girl. I had to break through postpartum a second time to be equipped with the tools I need to share with you so that you can conquer your setbacks.

As you commit to conquering your weaknesses, you'll develop a deeper relationship with God. The second breakdown led me to this break-through, so when he said the breakthrough was in me, I wholeheartedly knew that is what He meant without a doubt. Thank you, Father!

I've been telling people that this journey was not only physical but also spiritual. No one knew the depths of that. There were many things that I needed deliverance from and a lot of clarification during this fast.

My second birth brought me to another place of brokenness, loss, and confusion. He put me through a test of faith to grow spiritually, exercise my spiritual muscle, and extend that strength to enlighten others. In that time, I became stronger, and my strength was renewed. To understand this revelation, I will need to walk you through my second experience of postpartum depression.

I knew what direction my life was headed by having another un-planned pregnancy, and my only form of damage control was to prepare for the worst. Beyond surrendering my will to God, I felt it was time to entertain some of my gynecologist's referrals for therapy.

Show Up For Therapy: What Brings You In Today?

Finding a therapist during my second pregnancy was the best decision. That, in conjunction with fitness, opened the pathway to healing. Therapy is the greatest and most undervalued resource in the Black community.

Two months before Ever's birth, I attended my initial consult and never looked back. Based on my experience, I knew I would need to be proactive about ensuring that I was self-sufficient mentally after my pregnancy. I was terrified, but I knew it was an avenue I needed to explore.

It's funny because I was clueless about what to expect when I went into therapy. I was so paranoid and vulnerable, similar to when I expose myself during a Brazilian wax; I was uncertain if they knew me from social media and, if so, if my session remained confidential. Nevertheless, I had to do it naked and afraid.

Fortunately, the referral sheet consisted of a profile photo of each counselor. I found someone that looked as if we'd share the same interests. She was stunning. I said, "Hey, she may know a thing or two about life." She was poised and polished. She looked to be near my age, so I didn't look any further.

I would like to say that my discernment of character has aided me with grace throughout life. So I planned to tap into this divine power to determine if my therapist was the right fit. My appointment was at 12:00 p.m. on a Tuesday. I hesitantly waddled to the door and pressed the buzzer. When she opened the door, I immediately felt anxious, but I had already driven 45 minutes through traffic, so I had a quick mental self-talk and followed her to her couch of enlightenment.

Her hair was blonde in a top knot, and she wore the newest Fendi cowgirl boots. *I don't know if I can do this. This may be a little too distracting,* I thought. I wanted to focus on my internal transformation. I did not want to be reminded of the luxurious lifestyle I desired; I needed a neutral space for healing. If her Fendi boots were an indication of her wisdom, I felt I may be in a dilemma. I wondered if she was authentic or superficial. So, fully guarded, I proceeded with the session apprehensively because I didn't know if she was the surface person that I was trying to escape.

It's pretty standard for a therapist to do their normal spill. "Hi, I'm blah blah thank you for coming in." Then here comes the big kahuna question. "What brings you in today?" I drew a blank because I wanted to get straight to the meat of the situation. *Let's get straight to it. Why does everyone come to therapy, lady?*

After a deep breath, I regurgitated these words. "I am seven months pregnant, and I'm not sure what my future has in store. My grandfather is ill, and I'm not sure if he's going to make it. I'm about to have this baby, and I experienced postpartum depression in my previous pregnancy, so I don't know… I guess… I just want to leave here with peace and clarity."

I attended therapy for about three weeks before my grandfather passed away, four days before my baby shower, and ten days before my birthday. It was the worst birthday I'd had to date. Following this, I took a major unannounced break from social media to reflect. This gave me the solace that I needed to heal.

I resumed therapy closer to my delivery date when I found the strength to be transparent about my loss. The anxiety of giving birth again was surfacing slowly but surely. I was much more relaxed when my mom came into town. I vividly remember getting my last-minute things, purchasing clothes and strollers, decorating the baby's room, and completing my pre-partum tasks. Then came my tour of the hospital.

As I was heading into the parking deck of the facility, my phone rang. Reluctantly, I picked up the phone. It was an unknown contact number, a call from a mutual friend letting me know that a dear friend had passed away. I was at a loss for words. All I could do was cry and scream.

My mom was in the backseat, frantic because we had just lost my grandfather, and she didn't know if something was wrong with someone else in the family. I couldn't speak. My husband was driving, terrified and confused. I was screaming and crying uncontrollably. I was so sick (emotionally). Eventually, I had to say it. I had to say the words, and I had to deliver my baby the very next day.

I had no real time to process this loss. I just knew I couldn't be overly stressed because I had to have a healthy delivery, and God blessed me with just that. On December 10, 2019, I gave birth to a beautiful baby girl. Ever was 7 pounds and 13 ounces.

Although I was mourning, we were overjoyed. It's safe to say that I was in a different mental state when I gave birth to her. I was beyond grateful for a healthy delivery and was ready for war. I devoted my life to her protection and happiness. I wanted Ever to be healthy and was willing to do anything to ensure that.

Flex your spiritual muscle to reveal your strength."

TAE RENÉ

11

Faith Over Fear

Someone once asked me years ago how I was able to attend church weekly at a time in my life when nothing seemed to be working in my favor. I tried to break it down in terms that they would comprehend. I said you go to the gym, right? Well, the more consistent you are with your physical routine, the more you will develop muscle and become stronger. By going to church, I am exercising my spiritual muscle. This is how I maintain my spiritual strength.

Pain is a direct indicator of growth. In fitness, the higher the resistance, the more muscle you develop. You don't know when you'll need to use your muscles in life. You're just glad that they're conveniently present in times of need. Theoretically, this is how my spiritual muscles worked. I didn't know exactly when I would need it, but it was always something I relied upon.

Beyond character and physical results, when you simply don't have it in you, your spiritual strength will intercede and combat the thoughts of defeat deriving from your compromised mind on demand. We've conditioned our bodies to believe that only things that feel good are good for us. This can't be further from the truth.

During my second postpartum experience, I remained rooted in my faith. My faith sustained and guided me through days of sleep deprivation and unanticipated physical changes that sparked my recurring negative thoughts and feelings about myself. When I got on the scale after giving birth, I was 189 pounds. One would think that 60 pounds of weight gain resulted from carrying a 40-pound baby! Not so much. The baby was only eight pounds. Let's not add insult to injury here. Moving along.

*S*how Up Again?

The fact that I had already lost 60 lbs. once was my biggest motivation to do it again. I knew the pain to anticipate and the sacrifice it would require, which is also why I remained in therapy throughout my wellness journey. I knew what I was up against. The difference between now and then is that I was unstable, unhappy, and didn't have the financial security I have today. Don't judge. I was in my twenties. This time I was prepared and able to reference my previous postpartum experience. I found out how to show up for myself through faith and discipline. So, whether you're experiencing postpartum the first, second time around, or beyond, it's okay. I promise. You can overcome.

Many people don't know that this was my second time losing over 60 lbs. I had to become a different version of myself each time. What does this mean? Each time I had to tap into a higher discipline than the one I'd known previously. It meant working out on Saturdays and Sundays when most people slept in. It meant preparing my food at times when I was starving and driving past fast-food restaurants. The list goes on and on, but it was very much worth every single sacrifice. The elimination of your number one crutch can really impact your mental health. Trust me! I get it. I love to eat!

It is imperative that you know a few important things about me to better understand my journey. I LOVE FOOD. Potatoes, bread, and alcohol were my weakness. I am not an athlete, nor am I naturally thin. My genetic makeup is curvy, so naturally, I'm pretty thick. However, when you measure your success with previous victories, you can determine whether you're living at your fullest potential. At your core, you know when you are settling. All I wanted to do was be the best version of myself, not anyone else. There's a difference between being THE best and being YOUR best.

If you want to win this battle of the mind against the flesh, you must also know your strengths and weaknesses. With this knowledge, you will center your decisions on those that produce more favorable outcomes for your body. I recognized that I tend to make poor choices when I get anxious to subside the pressure. My environment easily influences me, and with this knowledge, I abstained from certain activities to reach my goal.

There have been numerous occasions when I've been out with friends and they'd look around the table and announce a round of shots following a rotation of spinach dip, calamari, and loaded fries. Oh, and please! Don't let it be Sunday brunch because the bottomless mimosas would be on the horizon. When embarking on a new lifestyle change, it's best to minimize the temptation.

Your environment is the key to your success, especially in the beginning phase of your journey. It will be challenging to avoid the lures of indulgence initially, especially fabulous dinner parties toasting to new endeavors every other week, such as we often do here in Atlanta. Thus it's imperative to also know what works for you.

As a results-oriented person, I do not like wasting time because, as we all know, time is money, honey! So, it didn't take much longer for my physical commitment to catch up with my renewed mentality. In reference to working out, my only focus was cardio and sculpting my abs which I learned when I was younger and interested in a workout regimen. However, that became all I knew and my go-to being a creature of habit. Recently, I've connected with an expert well-versed in fitness to help me focus on my goals.

Sometimes the force behind our bad habits is hard to recognize. Therapy ensured that everything always came to the surface. I became more comfortable confronting my feelings, even if there were things I didn't want to acknowledge. For example, there were areas in my life where I needed closure, such as forgiveness, letting go of the past, and defining myself beyond my external perception. My appetite began to grow for change. My therapist invited me to write out my thoughts and rekindle my relationship with my old journal.

I dug through the archives to give you a glimpse into my struggles. During my digging, I came across an old diet log of mine.

Here's a diet I attempted back in 2008. I had no idea of exactly what I was doing, but I had decided anything was better than where I was. The more I tried, the more I learned what to eat.

Crunches   Mon   Tues Wed.
  NR2   190   190 190
  NR2   190   190 200
         4 oz Jac Pints Crd

1. Thurs - Cereal, Tuna + crackers, tuna
   no lettuce + tomato, 2 bottles of water

2. Fri - English chicken sandwich, x Ham
   Ham Apple Juice 1 bott of water

3. Sat - 2 bowls of cereal, no H2O 2 Aunt
   Made

4. Sun - Nana's open House eating to us
   till 8:00 😠 Ensure salad a piece fried chicken, a
   small dish of macaroni Ensure twigs of bread, piece of
   roasted no H2O, that's it!

5. Mon - bowl of cereal + sandwich 2 pieces

My Diet

"*Authenticity is
always in style.*"

TAE RENÉ

12

Post to Be

The kind of showing up that exceeds your expectations is putting in the work daily, going to the gym, and being intentional about what you consume. The music, food, TV, conversations, absolutely everything you consume are factors in your overall success. I slept better at night, fully assured that I woke up to a better version of myself each day. Before I knew it, I had lost 5 lbs., 10lbs., 15 lbs., 20 lbs., and then 50 lbs. I exceeded my weight loss goal just as I had during my first postpartum experience. All I had to do was keep showing up.

It didn't always happen as planned, though. I would often set deadlines and find that I hadn't met them. I never will forget my birthday on October 14th. I had already lost 30 pounds, but my goal was to be at my prepartum weight by my birthday, as I would have been ten months post-partum. I figured sure! That's plenty of time to get there. I stood on the scale at 143, extremely disappointed, but I didn't allow that to deter me. I decided to take my transparency to social media.

taetv I had so many reservations about posting this photo because:

A. I never wear my arms out because I feel that they are obnoxiously large lol (personal don't judge me)

B. I was going to use my Picasso Facetune skills to edit both pics but I decided to share my personal growth 🙃

C. I appreciate all of the love and support I've received on my fitness journey BUT I am still a work in progress anddd I'm not done yet!

I had a baby 10 months ago. I lost 47 lbs! The right high-waisted pants will have me looking snatched. However, there's some postpartum realness beneath that waist line and I'm actually still swollen.

Loving myself at all phases of this process means living in truth. This is my second postpartum weight loss experience and let me say for the record that IT WAS harder this time 😫 almost as hard as having the baby lol. Like seriously, but I deserve it and you all deserve this transparency because the last thing that I'm trying to do is give anyone false hope!

2,598 likes

Comments

Authenticity is fading in my community (beauty) so I wanted to spread some light and love on the topic of physical wellness by sharing my reality. You too can have your cake and eat it too when you have realistic expectations 🥂 #cheers

Swipe for the real teal 1st pic is retouched 😅 (IG vs. real life)

DISCLAIMER: LET ME ALSO SAY that this is how I feel in this moment and should I decide to proceed with any cosmetic reconstruction in the future, please don't be disappointed. I am still celebrating where I am today 👏

Social Media Transparency

Under my post, it read:

I had so many reservations about posting this photo because:

A. *I never wear my arms out because I feel that they are obnoxiously large lol (personal don't judge me)*
B. *I was going to use my Picasso Face tune skills to edit both pics, but I decided to share my personal growth*
C. *I appreciate all of the love and support I've received on my fitness journey, BUT I am still a work in progress, and I'm not done yet!*

I had a baby ten months ago. I lost 47 lbs.! The right high-waisted pants will have me looking snatched. However, there's some postpartum realness beneath that waistline, and I'm actually still swollen.

Loving myself at all phases of this process means living in truth. This is my second postpartum weight loss experience and let me say for the record that IT WAS harder (physically) this time almost as hard as having the baby, lol. Like seriously, I deserve it, and you all deserve this transparency because the last thing that I'm trying to do is give anyone false hope!

Authenticity is fading in my community (beauty), so I wanted to spread some light and love on the topic of physical wellness by sharing my reality. You too can have your cake and eat it too when you have realistic expectations #che

Swipe for the real tea! 1ˢᵗ pic is retouched (IG vs. real life)

DISCLAIMER: LET ME ALSO SAY that this is how I felt at this moment, and should I decide to proceed with any cosmetic reconstruction in the future, please don't be disappointed. I am still celebrating where I am today

This was one of my highest-performing posts. I received so many comments and positive feedback. There were women from all walks of life sharing their stories. I was overcome with so much compassion. It motivated me. Women shared photos of their postpartum bodies, and they thanked me for having the courage to be vocal about my experience.

It was comforting to know that I wasn't alone, specifically within the

Black community of women. The issue with postpartum depression and weight loss in the Black community is simply the lack of awareness. We can't repair what we don't identify as broken. What's broken as a result of childbirth is our spirits and minds. The body is a physical manifestation of that dysfunction. This made me realize that we need more love.

I was elated that many women began their wellness journeys and kept me updated on their progress. It was an honor to help them reach their goals. My mom even took her diet more seriously. She started cooking healthier at home, and she lost 20 pounds. Lo and behold, everywhere I looked, I could see many focused women changing their lives by showing up for themselves.

I continued to share my before and after photos on social media, which had an upward domino effect on my recovery. The more transparent I became, the more feedback I received. The more feedback I received, the more effort I put forth. This truly reinforced my mission of helping others realize their potential. Aside from fitness, I intend to share all areas of breakthrough in my life. I am eager to remind all women that they are worthy, strong, and able to overcome hardship and provide clear, actionable guidance to empower them on their path to happier, healthier lives.

The act of motherhood hasn't been forgotten, but the woman behind the role suffers and is often overlooked. Aside from being the vessel of life (literally), we're human beings that need reassurance and support. Strangers, friends, and family alike should aid in shining light in our direction. It's a dire need for women at large.

"Criticism and confidence can't live in the same space."

TAE RENÉ

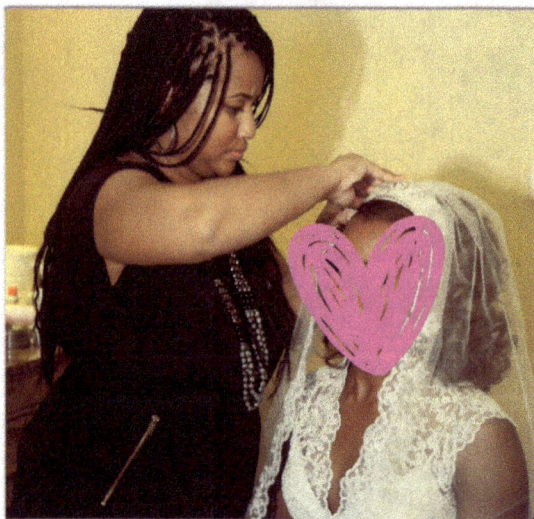

My Postpartum Appearance

13

Crop Top Conformity

I dreaded the moment of revealing my postpartum body to friends and colleagues. Contrary to the rising demand for real bodies, there was an even bigger lack of suitable attire. I found myself in an all too familiar position scurrying through my wardrobe for the perfect attire. It was déjà vu, reminiscent of my first work experience after the birth of my eldest daughter, Ella.

A client of mine was getting married in Florida when Ella was two months old. She didn't trust anyone else with her hair and makeup. I was honored that she entrusted me. However, I was still fearful of my postpartum appearance while traveling for the first time after birth.

Here we are yet again. Baby Ever was just 4 months old, and a friend of mine was getting married in Mexico. I had just a few weeks to prepare for her wedding. It was not the ideal time to reveal my postpartum body. In the most proactive fashion, I decided to order some nice clothes online.

As I searched the internet repeatedly, I wondered why there were hardly any full-length shirts. Not to mention it was spaghetti strap and spandex central. My oh my! After scrolling for hours, I decided to leave my home and physically go to a nearby boutique. To my disbelief, there were absolutely no full-length shirts.

"Ma'am?" I asked the associate.

"Can I help you?"

"Do you carry full-length t-shirts?"

"If we do, they would be folded up on the table there," she responded.

"And do you carry full-length blouses?" I inquired.

"Oh, no, we don't."

Wow, ok. So there is absolutely no merchandise on the planet that caters to regular bodies. Great!

I skimmed through rack after rack.

No, I need a bra on. I can't wear this. Omg, my FUPA will be the center of attention. In case you didn't know FUPA is known as the "fatty upper pubic area". My thoughts continued.

I cannot with this sleeveless number. How am I going to wear my waist trainer under this? I love this shirt. Why is it only 3/4 worth of fabric?

I searched and searched only for nothing to avail. Trying to find flattering clothes to wear was like fighting an uphill battle these days.

It was like finding a needle in a haystack. Then, it suddenly clicked. There's no wonder so many women will get plastic surgery now. There are no more regular clothes available that suit our bodies! I think the rise in Brazilian butt lifts, also known as BBLs, and abdominoplasty has a lot to do with the fact that it's hard to find a full-length shirt in today's era.

If, like most mothers, you suffer from physical trauma such as diastase recti, finding fashions that don't enhance those features is atypical. We must take all these things into consideration. Is the waistline high enough? Can I wear my Spanx with it? Can I wear a waist trainer with it? Will my bra strap show? Lord knows I don't need these saggy boobs saddling in the chest cups of this top. The understatement of frustration can't even begin to describe how I felt. It triggered me, reminding me of my first postpartum shopping experience.

My judgment remained. I did not want to wear any clothing that clung to my body. Surely, I saw my progress, but I still wasn't quite there. In a world of mom-shaming, body-shaming, and postpartum-snapback shaming, I simply decided to put my best effort forth but keep it tasteful.

Desperate and feeling defeated, I grabbed the biggest t-shirt and black tights that I could find.

I had to find comfort in knowing that this would be a process. You see, after my first childbirth, I was 25; hence certain body parts snapped back. It may not have been my stomach, but my legs snapped back for sure. This time "Oh my! That is not what happened. If I had to smooth the cellulite of my legs via that picture app again, I was going to lose it!

You know how some Christians have the infamous testimony, "Praise God I don't look like what I've been through." Well, that was not the case for me. Some areas of my body looked like what it had gone through.

"Sometimes you have to put your big-girl panties on."

TAE RENÉ

14

The Postpartum Pandemic

The trip to Mexico revealed that feelings and thoughts are real but do not always tell the truth. No one said a word about my exterior. Upon returning to the United States with frozen breast milk in tow, an announcement was made that we were in a global pandemic, followed by the chaos of quarantining, home-schooling, and no alone time. I felt my mental and physical health progress reversing. I hit a plateau that I never could have anticipated.

Thank God for my virtual counseling sessions. My bougie counselor was almost my best friend, but she was the kind of friend who listened to your problems without exposing any of her own. When building a relationship, it's important to share your lows and highs and be vulnerable together, in my opinion. I had to get comfortable with knowing that the relationship with my counselor had a different dynamic.

She made me feel normal in my postpartum recovery. She shared that she had children of her own and that postpartum was something I should take seriously. Sometimes I just wanted to share some wild and crazy stories to see her response and if she was relatable, but she never compromised her poise.

Eventually, I came to terms with the fact that she is the bougie friend who knows all of your secrets that never has a hair out of place. Either way, she allowed me to go on my rants and vent from time to time with intention, of course. Her mantra was being mindful of our thoughts and actions… blah blah blah. I kid, I kid. All jokes aside, she was always understanding, and without our weekly meetings, I'm unsure if I would have survived the pandemic.

It was time for my second postpartum checkup when the doctor asks if you are experiencing depressing thoughts. My natural response was no, even though I had previously experienced this "low" feeling.

"Do you think you're experiencing postpartum?"

"Probably so."

"We can prescribe you some medications to help you cope."

I didn't want to become dependent on medication. Let me clarify. I am not pill shaming. I just didn't want the risk of my baby consuming the medication through excreted breast milk.

I told her, "No, thank you."

"Are you sure?" she asked.

"Yes, I'll just do what I know when I'm able to do that."

"Okay, and what might that be?"

"I'm going to work out and pray."

Taken aback, she glanced up at me and said, "That's great and good luck; if you find that you aren't progressing, please do not hesitate to come back and see us."

"Thanks!"

I removed my paper robe as she exited, donned my postpartum panties, nursing bra, and XXL sweatsuit, and confidently headed out of the door.

"Never underestimate a Black woman on a mission."

TAE RENÉ

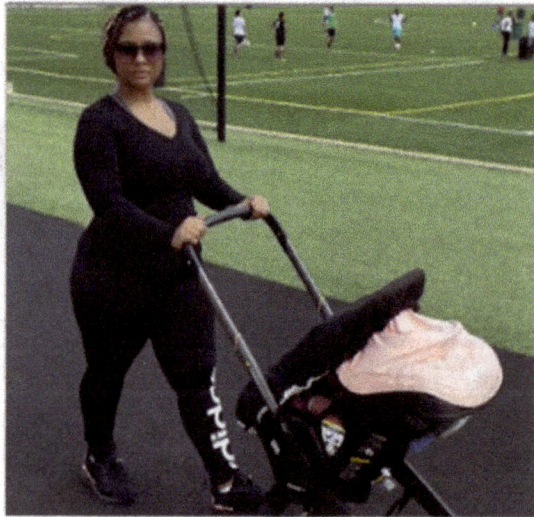

I am " Black" on Track

15

"Black" on Track

"I'm uncomfortable where I am physically, and I feel it's manifesting in other areas of my life," I told my therapist. "I feel like everyone sees me differently. I'm not even sure that my husband is still attracted to me."

"Are you sure these are not just your feelings?" my therapist asked. "You know, oftentimes when we feel a way about ourselves, we project those feelings onto others, and it's really just a reflection of our own opinions."

She said, "Okay, gradually, you have to do something about it."

But I wasn't ready. I hadn't worked out in a few months. The last time I exercised was in preparation for my friend's wedding. In the days ahead, my commitment to therapy truly helped me develop a realistic pace in rediscovering my ambition and confronting the things that burdened me.

After being locked down for months during the pandemic with a newborn, On August 14th, 2020, I decided to stop making excuses. I found a neighborhood track and went to work. This was my first attempt to run outdoors; if I'm fully transparent, the process didn't initially feel very productive.

At 4 foot 11 inches and 180 lbs., I decided to step outside to run. I remember feeling heavy, like my ankle might twist if my leg landed wrong. Parts of my body shook in places that I had never known existed. I felt like I looked foolish, and it didn't help that I was surrounded by people in their fitness prime.

BUT I had the support of my husband, my babies, and I knew I could do it. I had done it before! I also wanted my oldest baby girl to watch me evolve so that she, too, could know that you can get through anything. Yep, I had to bring my kids and hubby in tow in case of a nursing emergency, as I was still breastfeeding. My girls were always in close proximity.

Although I didn't know if I would get through that first mile, my hopes were high. Their eyes watching me outweighed every insecurity I had. I turned on Map, my favorite fitness app, to track my run and tuned into my GO Hard or GO home S.U.F.Y. (Show Up for Yourself) playlist featuring a curated list of raps I've collected over four years that get me pumped and pushed through.

I didn't care how foolish I looked. I channeled my inner beast. I was determined to complete that mile whether I had to stop and walk for a little while or not. But it turns out curvy girls can run too. Although my curvy girl phase was short-lived, I had to represent, and that's what I kept reinforcing in my mind as I blazed through those two half-mile laps.

I have a few songs on the S.U.F.Y. playlist that help me bring it home during a run.

I got it done, and I didn't even have to stop. My oldest baby girl was cheering me on. My husband gave me a nice pat on the tush, and I was feeling myself all over again—all 180 pounds of me.

I ran on that track religiously for at least four months from that point onward. Upon the gym reopening (I should elaborate on how I couldn't work out during the pandemic), I was one of the first ones in the building when the gym reopened. Working out had become the release again that I had once known. When I finally posted a before and after of me running on the track, the video went viral and had over 100,000 likes and 1.2 million views. The love was so inspirational.

"You don't have to be great to start, but you do have to start to be great!"

ZIG ZIGLAR

16

Marathon-Minded

Of course, our body gets accustomed to our workout routine. I've experienced this on more than one occasion. However, this time around, it was unacceptable. I decided to take matters into my own hands. I had reached a plateau in my weight when I was approached for a brand partnership with a Black-owned juice bar. So, I did their 7-day juice challenge. This was a business that could actually benefit my health, so I committed. Not knowing what to expect, I dove right in. I felt this was an opportunity I didn't want to pass up.

The Perfect Pear Juice Bar was generous in knowledge and health insights. Not only did they guide me in how to successfully complete the juice cleanse, but they were also always available to answer all my questions throughout the process. The juice cleanses consisted of four juices I was allowed to drink daily, containing only fruits, vegetables, and water for seven days. Though I was warned to only attempt three days, being more than ready, I committed to seven. I couldn't believe the number that I was staring at on the scale on day 7. Then I added three more days.

To prepare myself for the cleanse, I decided the best way to succeed was to transition my eating habits and consume all fruits and vegetables for one full day. It had been so long since I juiced. I wanted to ensure that I was prepared. It worked! I was hardly hungry when I started the "Waist

SnatcHer Cleanse." In order to avoid relapse moments, I drank plenty of water in between.

This was a spiritual fast; it helped me regain control of my body. To commit to this, I took my mental shift a step further. This felt beyond me, like something beyond all that I've ever done, but I was tired of my weight fluctuating. This was the healthiest weight that I'd been since my 20s. When I reached my 120-lb weight goal, I said, "Okay, maybe I will share my journey." Then a rebuttal arose. "No, what if you gain the weight right back?" It wasn't until I actually maintained the weight that I could be confident in sharing my story.

The greatest benefit of seeing this process through is that I could think quicker and move faster. Also, since I prayed throughout this process, I felt more centered. I feel that I have actually improved as a human being. When you think about who you can become in the process, and if you have the will to do that, you can do anything. There's no limit to what you can do.

What you resist implementing in your lifestyle persists. Therefore, focus on your evolution, not limitation. Don't think about what you can't eat. Don't think about what you can no longer have. I'm a firm believer in only speaking what you want. Whether you believe it or not, when words come out of your mouth, you give life to them. The power of life and death lies in the tongue. What you give life, you get in return.

Adopt a Marathon Mentality

Show yourself you are a champion. Make yourself a believer! The reason you don't believe in yourself is because you're a tough critic and actions speak louder to you than words in your world. In the same way you would want a dating candidate to prove that they're worthy of your time, apply the same strategy to yourself. It's okay, girl! You have standards so high that you don't even believe yourself until you show up and prove it! This mentality confirms exactly where you're supposed to be.

Post to Be

The evolution of catfishing has become the greatest digital scam in the world. Trust me. As a makeup artist, I've been considered an accomplice in such deception. Who are we trying to impress on social media? Most of the time, it's ourselves. It's just unfortunate the lengths we'll go to impress or lure others in. The impression we give others is essentially what impresses us. Think about how you strive to be perceived; successful, happy, and well-balanced. In a culture of photo editing, advanced shapewear, non-invasive body sculpting, accessible plastic surgery, and capping (as the kids call lying) at an all-time high, the pursuit of natural weight loss has seemingly lost its value.

Sculpt Me

Who really needs plastic surgery when you have access to photo-editing apps? I can take my waist from 30 inches to 24 in one pinch. I can make my boobs appear larger, my butt bigger, and my hips wider. You'll be looking at Jessica Rabbit by the time I'm done. And that's exactly what I'll be, a fictional character, not my true self.

People are so caught up in the "ideal" image on social media that they forget what a real woman looks like. In desperate measures, people are leaving the country to undergo bariatric procedures such as gastroplasty. Presently, in the United States, there is a weight requirement to have this operation performed. This is a great procedure for those who are challenged beyond their natural ability to lose weight. However, some traveled overseas and have been only 40 pounds overweight or less. The surgery consists of rerouting the gastrointestinal tract, minimizing the number of calories you can consume. Whistle-blow much? In efforts to keep everyone safe, absolutely!

Nevertheless, passports are flooded with entry stamps from the East as people are risking their lives getting the procedure for half the price. To be considered a candidate in America for gastroplasty, your weight would have to exceed your ideal weight past 80-100 pounds with a Body mass index of 35-39 and a chronic health condition related to obesity. In addition to committing to making long-term lifestyle changes, you'd have to agree to long-term post-operative care.

Make no mistake. I'm not surgery-shaming as I'm no stranger to plastic surgery. While writing this book, I'm currently in the last phases of augmentation mammoplasty recovery. I underestimated the value of my elbows! I haven't been able to lift my arms for weeks. I decided to finally get my breasts done.

When all of my peers were going through puberty, circa early millennia, my petite little frame resisted. Hips, butt, and breasts were simply not the highlight of my body. I'd like to imagine it was my innocent smile. Although I was accustomed to the void, I couldn't help but recognize it as a physical debacle when I reached my twenties.

I discovered a padded bra artifice that carried me for a decade and some change. You would have never known I'd lacked, but when I had children, oh my! It just wasn't the same. Can you imagine that something you're already insecure about worsening postpartum?

After nursing my two children, the sight of my breasts was distressing. My left breast was significantly longer than my right. Yes, I said longer because those babies needed a little assistance in the lift department. They simply hung, and even when I put on a bra, they just saddled inside the bra. I could literally look in my chest and see the rippled skin sagging together. I would joke seriously but make light that they must have resembled elephant testicles with an added areola.

One time at an event, I undressed in front of my mother, who was in the room trying to help me decide on my dress, and she just busted out in laughter.

"What's so amusing?"

"My poor baby. I know I don't have any breasts, but they've never looked that bad."

"Geez, mom, really?" I muttered.

Weeks later, I was exploring my options at Tailor Made Looks, a plastic surgery center in the heart of the prestigious Buckhead Atlanta. Dr. Berhane made it clear that my abdominal trauma was from weight loss and that I had excessive loose skin. He assured me, however, that my issues could be corrected. I wasn't ready for abdominoplasty, but I was open to his suggestions for augmentation.

I was so nervous on the day of the procedure. Never in a million years did I imagine having an operation, no matter how dissatisfied I was with my breasts. I was afraid, but I was ready. Fear would not stop me. Weeks later, when my surgical tape was removed at my follow-up visit, I felt like a new woman. I was amazed at my results. However, you should do your own research and consult your physician if you are considering getting a surgical procedure. Not to mention that the results may vary.

I contemplated long and hard about whether I would move further into my weight loss journey and get abdominoplasty. My stomach looks exactly as my breasts had pre-operation. I told myself I would do everything within my absolute power to naturally enhance my body, and I did. But people don't realize that transformational weight loss also comes with a price—stretched skin.

I also suffer from what is known as diastasis recti. This is when your left and right abdominal muscles have separated as a result of giving birth. This, combined with the aftermath of weight loss, wasn't a pretty sight. Hence your stomach appears pudgy, or you have the infamous pooch that 2 out of 3 mothers experience. It's especially common for women that have undergone Cesarean operations. I underwent two cesareans to give birth to my babies. High-waist me, please! In case you're not that cool, it's kind of a thing to take a noun and convert it to a verb to add a dramatic effect to a statement.

Ironically, my recovery time from plastic surgery and a covid recovery in my family have resulted in a few added pounds as I've not been able to go to the gym. So, believe it or not, I will be revisiting my own method right along with you. I've gained five pounds! I also recommend not fully relying on the scale but paying close attention to how your clothes fit and measuring yourself occasionally to keep track of your waist loss in inches.

Upon completing my juice cleanse, I committed to a vegan lifestyle. I was consuming only plant-based foods, mostly 80% raw. I was very lean during this time. However, I did not consume potatoes of any kind.

Check out this photo gallery snapshot of my vegan diet.

Visual Diet

Honestly, there is no one way to lose weight, and not everything works for everyone. I became a pescopaleoplantbasedtarian. Just kidding! Ostroveganism sounded tempting, as well as lacto-ovo vegetarianism. Maybe I'm a lacto-ovo pescatarian. Is this too much? It sounds like some type of foot fungal diagnosis. Ostroveganism is a diet that consists of a full vegan diet and includes mussels, clams, scallops, and oysters. Lacto-ovo means that you entertain some eggs in your diet. I think the closest food clique I would be affiliated with would be lacto-ovo pescatarian. At times, I eat fish, eggs, and dairy.

Here's the thing, diets have gotten so complicated these days. You would think there's an initiation process to even get started. Why do these dietary categories sound like gangs and religions? So I took it upon myself to create my own version of a diet. I've created an MGC diet. Contrary to the "See" food diet where you eat everything you see, I'd like to define the MGC diet as the "Make Good Choices" diet. Lately, I've found that between running errands, writing this book, and producing content for a new show, sometimes you just have to make the best choices from what you have.

Here is what has been effective for me. I consume my largest meal earlier in the day. This way, I will have the remainder of the day for it to metabolize and digest, whereas when you consume your larger meals later in the day, it metabolizes slower because people tend to be less active in the evenings. Each day the average person burns about 1800 calories with absolutely no activity whatsoever. With that in mind, it's safe to say that it's not exactly required to work out to lose weight, as 70% of weight loss results from what you eat. I also ensure that I drink plenty of water and snack to avoid aggressive hunger spells throughout the day.

Here's another tip: Take it one day at a time. If you're a soda drinker, eliminate soda from your diet and keep everything else consistent on day one. On Day 2, you can take it a step further and eliminate fast food and sodas. This can also go from week one to week two and vice versa. Keep track of your progress because it motivates you to continue to be persistent. Don't forget those small victories. Those small victories are major wins.

I can't help but testify that as you look back on your life, I'm almost certain that you can recall experiencing hard times when you had no idea how you were going to get through, but you survived. It may have been involuntary, but you outlived it and are still here. You know where I'm going with this, right? If you've endured the absolute hardest phases of your life, I know you can survive a few diet modifications to achieve the body of your dreams.

Semantically, when you break down the word, achieve what do you see? I'll tell you what you see. You see a "chief." This means that your success results from the dominion you've taken over your body. You're the chief of your progress and achievement. You're in charge. No one else can tell your body what to do. This means that you have to take full ownership of where you are in this journey or where you are not.

How to Maintain Your Weight Loss

As much as we aim to reach our weight loss goals, we must fight to maintain them. However, this discipline has become second nature, just like the weight loss process. It's not difficult to sustain. I often hear that the hardest part of weight loss is keeping the weight off.

I encourage you to avoid "fad diets" and diets that make you lose weight fast, such as the Lemonade diet, a special drink composed of lemons, maple syrup, and cayenne pepper accompanied by a saltwater flush day and night. There's also something known as the military diet. These diets limit you to a restricted calorie intake per day. The idea is that you eat the restricted foods for three days and return to your regular diet for the next four. The diet is high in protein and low in carbohydrates, calories, and fat.

I've tried the lemonade diet once, and I'll say that it was effective but a temporary weight loss method. As soon as I began eating solid foods, the weight packed right back on, and that could be exactly what it's designed for—short-term results. Sometimes short-term results are important! It is that serious in certain circumstances, such as a wedding, vacation, or photoshoot. Your weight is guaranteed to fluctuate using short term weight loss methods.

People complain to me all the time.

"Tae, everyone is not like you. Everybody doesn't have the same discipline to lose weight."

A lot of my friends tell me. I'm not even going to contest. You see? I agree; however, I also agree because they're making the conscious decision not to. They're prioritizing something else. Indecision is still a decision. If you chose to delight in chicken alfredo and buttery garlic bread, you simply prioritized your desire for taste over your desire for physical wellness.

All habits, good or bad, lead to results. Whether you're being intentional or chancing life, something is happening as a result. You can choose to be the pilot of that venture or simply be a passenger along for the ride.

Consistently making poor eating choices results in weight gain and can compromise your health in the long run. However, it's just as easy making a healthy choice as it is making an unhealthy choice. You must control your eating habits.

I'm very flattered that people think I activate a superpower when I eat clean and work out. However, I'm just choosing to show up for myself in this way. I reclaimed power over my body and maintained dominion because I have shown up and never left.

What about cheat days, you may wonder? I don't recommend cheat days early in your journey because your mind is still vulnerable. My goal is to ultimately recondition and change your desires. If you continue backtrack-sampling from the former version of yourself, you'll eventually fall back into the habit of entertaining those foods. I'll speak for myself in terms of addiction. It takes 90 days to break an addiction. In the past, when I considered allowing myself a cheat day, I took a small bit of a

French fry, then I ate the whole fry, another fry, and eventually, I ate the whole box of fries and totally relapsed.

Here's another common excuse that many people say, "I'm trying, but it's not working." Oh, it is working, but you're not. I hate to be gut-wrenchingly honest, but someone has to do the hard stuff! Otherwise, you won't hold yourself accountable.

If you are in control of your own body, then trying is unacceptable. You're either doing it, or you're not. This is what separates those who want to show up and those who want to remain where they are. Your best self awaits you, and all you have to do is the work.

"Your reflection is your truth."

TAE RENÉ

17

Representation Matters

Since when has fashion become figure-specific? Maybe I'm having a "you don't know what you have until it's gone moment." I wasn't concerned about postpartum clothing options prepartum. Well, sometimes it takes an experience to make you aware. There's nothing wrong with being the change that you want to see. Surely mom bods (bodies) aren't on the priority list when it comes to inventory.

After paying tuition, car notes, mortgages, and student loans, moms are the ones with the dern money! If you ask me, there is a niche that has been forgotten in this world when it pertains to body image. When you think about it, there's a section for plus, petite, and maternity, but what about the most popular category that is, "I'm not at my ideal weight, hide my back rolls, and fupa from the right high forward-tilting camera angle, I look amazing," postpartum body? I'm talking about post-nursing breasts and all! This body type has yet to be celebrated, let alone the diastasis recti, "oatmeal pie," wrinkle tummy, stretch-marked mama.

The void in representation just got real, folks! Show me an average-body-sized woman or any woman for that matter with the honorable mark of motherhood- the diastasis recti, stretch marks, and saggy boobs. Can you recall a film, runway show, or publication where it's been featured? Better yet, show me a hot-single woman gracing a cover bearing these marks of glory. Do people talk about it at all? Why not, might you ask? Have you ever heard that conversation?

If I'd been aware that the reflection of my body represented the majority of the women in my age group, postpartum depression would not have invaded my life the way it had years ago. Let's get to the root of the problem. What caused the glamorization of high-profile breasts, flawless skin, thin waists, and obnoxious hips? Who created this prototype that is merely a facade of women?

Why don't we show our real bodies? Why is our post-mom abdomen something we hide well, at least I hid it, for a long time? We have our own category. When you can show me an ad with a woman in a bikini wearing those glorious marks of birth, I will know that there has been a shift in the perspective of beauty. As long as a woman is confident enough, she should have the same opportunities as a runway model.

From the distressed skin to the wear and tear of a woman after birth are noble wounds! If anything, it should be put on a pedestal. We are a forgotten tribe, a deliberate extinction that should be celebrated instead of inhibited. Have we been inadvertently conditioned to hate our bodies by the common public? If representation matters, where is ours? One may argue that we weren't denied. We were just not included. Omittance is not necessarily rejection, but it is, in fact, nonrecognition. It's time for us to reclaim our space. Well, proclaim one.

Time Matters

Organization is a very easy way to ensure you are successful on your wellness journey. While pursuing my personal transformation, I've managed my days with the utmost effort. This includes performing daily chores and mommy tasks and overseeing my work schedule. Meal prepping is the ultimate challenge. Although it didn't work for me, I ensured that I made time to shop for groceries, have them delivered, and prepare daily meals for my family.

Time management is essential to your wellness plans. Knowing how much time you have to dedicate to your wellness will help you become accountable, eradicate excuses, and maintain the discipline to effectively manage family, career, and self-care. My wellness plan included picking up my children from school, ensuring my family ate dinner, and completing my evening workout. Your plan may differ from mine. As you embark on this journey, creating and respecting your boundaries is imperative to achieve the results you deserve.

My SUFY Sisters Matter

You may be wondering, why are you sharing all this information on how you've met your weight loss goals? Sis, you're giving the game away. Now your competition can one-up you. Not exactly, because unfortunately for most, even given all this insight, they simply won't apply it. I know, I know, that's not you, though.

Can you count how many times you've researched a makeup look or recipe to duplicate only to get halfway in and want to throw the brush or spoon? I know that I have. Your efforts reflect your passion. There's no way that if I were passionate enough about a subject, I would give up! I would keep trying until I got it right.

There are over five different weight loss strategies mentioned in this book:

1. Utilizing a calorie counting app
2. The Limited Carb Diet
3. The Vegan Diet
4. MGC Diet
5. The Juice Cleanse
6. Intermittent Fasting

If you're not interested in logging your food for the day, then stick with Make Good Choices, carb-curving, and intermittent fasting. Follow the tips for consuming your water and keeping snacks, and I'm certain you will see progress.

My Sister's Business

As I mentioned, I am about my sister's business, meaning that if there was any way that I could use my talents and experience to show them their power, I am all for it. You know how they say if you can do something for free, that's where you will find your purpose? My passion is freeing confined minds and aiding them in expanding to their unlimited potential. It's not the process I love but the product that brings me joy. I did not discover that until just now in writing this very sentence, which brings me to how this book came about. I've accessed a power I didn't know I possessed and decided to share my experience to help you reach your goals. This book has been enlightening for me, and I hope it is for you.

My Heart Behind It All

This brings me circa 2008, when I discovered the power of beauty and decided to make a career of it and educate others on the topic. I had no guidance when I first moved to Atlanta. There were no women in sight to look at me and say, "Hey, let me help this poor girl be the best that she can be."

I was invisible and, like many young girls, was willing to do what it took to reach my goals. In retrospect, my journey has been more about what I have given than what I've received. With what I've received, I'm honored to give.

There were countless doors that I was turned away from because I didn't "look the part," and at the time, I didn't have the budget to have someone help me level up. So guess what? I picked up a makeup brush and a flat iron and changed the trajectory of my journey, not to mention a few opinions along the way.

You will encounter distractions on your path to becoming the ULTIMATE you, but that's expected. You're walking into uncharted territory here. My former approach to transforming women was from the outside in. This time it's from the inside out. You will also encounter many people who don't believe in you, but you have to believe in God and His purpose.

Once I mastered beauty, it was a wrap! I used my gifts to show other women their confidence in hopes that, in turn, they would go out into the world and pay it forward by exemplifying confidence in ways that are life-changing for other women. When I say that I'm about my sister's business, it means that I'm about my S.U.F.Y. sisters' growth. I'm about her internal success and willingness to instill and reaffirm the ideas of wealth, abundance, and courage.

Thus, 12 years later, I want to help you transform your mind. The freedom of living your truth is beyond gratifying. You'll find that every time you set a goal, you crush it and set a bigger one. This is more about the internal work that benefits the external. Not only am I about my sister's business, but I'm also about my community's business. When I empower women with tools for growth and knowledge, they can take leaps into spaces they never knew how to inhabit.

I thrive on witnessing the transformation of a woman, how she goes from bare and vulnerable with me to glamorous, empowered, and assertive. She is ready to overcome adversity and conquer the world. My initial armor was a curling iron and a makeup brush. But now, it's knowledge, discipline, and my disposition against limits. You can achieve everything you imagine and beyond. This is my newly adopted philosophy.

*S*tay Inspired

I use a strategic approach when following people on social media. I follow athletes, entertainers, stay-at-home moms, and influencers who exhibit discipline, tenacity, and consistency. In addition, I subscribed to healthy food profiles for recipes and trainers who embodied health as a lifestyle. This is one way I stayed motivated and on track to reach my goals.

I also highly suggest utilizing the power of visualization and your imagination to achieve your goals. This may sound a little bit obsessive, but I have a Pinterest board labeled "Bawdy" for all of my body inspiration. If you do not find pictures of inspiration on Pinterest, you can upload your own images and post them. I'm no Pinterest expert; however, I know how to do the minimum. When you create it, share your board with me! I would love to see it!

"It's about progression, not perfection."

TAE RENÉ

18

Imperfection to Progression

"I'm okay, hydrated, and not hungry. My kids are at school, and I'm off today. Now what?" In the past, this would have been an indulgent moment of fine dining and overpriced cocktails followed by repetitive weight gain and excessive workouts to shed the pounds. It was the counterproductivity for me; it kept me on the hamster wheel of weight loss.

An idle mind is the enemy's playground. How many times have you heard this? When you fail to plan, you plan to fail. There have been times when I didn't know what to do. You will find this very often at the beginning of your journey because now your awareness has shifted. I planned for this moment so I wouldn't fail. I was intentional about being prepared for unexpected moments and downtime. Since I know this is a vulnerability of mine, I created a list of tasks that I could apply to my goals.

I always referenced a list of goals that I call my "S.U.F.Y. Power List." This would be a list of things that I hadn't achieved, such as writing this book, for instance, or researching a new product. I found myself being the most productive at this time. My pursuit of showing up for myself created a habitual proactive beast within me that I had yet to meet. I gave my attention to the things that directly aided me in making my dreams come true. No matter what you do, as long as you are proactive and executing positive actions, you will unlock the universal principle of reaping what you sow, which is LAW.

I love mirror moments because you see who you are and how far you've grown. You can appreciate yourself for showing up and see the reflection you are proud of. Your reflection is your truth.

I want you to take a moment to write the goals you want to achieve.

1. _____
2. _____
3. _____
4. _____
5. _____
6. _____
7. _____
8. _____
9. _____
10. _____

Now create a list of action tasks for each goal from beginning to end.

1. _____
2. _____
3. _____
4. _____
5. _____
6. _____
7. _____
8. _____
9. _____
10. _____

This is your S.U.F.Y. Power List. This will keep you on track. So, when you're thinking about what to do and have idle time, assess your list, and take action. Little by little, you will scratch off every duty and reach your ultimate goals.

I once told a popular influencer I wanted to become a millionaire. She looked at me and said, "Girl! At least make it two." This became motivation for me. She had already reached her million-dollar milestone. She pushed me to not only dream big but bigger. This is why conversing with like-minded people who want to see you win is important.

You must be willing to do whatever it takes to reach your goals, not just in weight loss but in life. You have to map it out and then get straight to work. Make your success non-negotiable in all areas. The sooner you get to work, the faster you learn what works for you and what doesn't. You can always use life's feedback to tailor your experience to suit your goals.

"The power of life and death lies within the tongue."
—Proverbs 18:21

It's very seldom that I can actively pursue my goals without a disruptive imposter syndrome attack. One of the greatest challenges while becoming an author and advocate was imposter syndrome. I had thoughts of being underqualified, undeserving of success, and the inability to accomplish my goals. Constantly, I was conflicted between self-perception and the way others perceived me.

I almost talked myself out of writing a book that would be transformative for myself and others! Even now, as I'm typing. Who do I think I am? What makes you think people want to listen to you? You're not an author. *All these voices.* In like spirit, these voices once said, who are you kidding? You're so big. Even if you lose five pounds, nobody will notice because you'll still be fat. You're going running? Pick the loosest outfit to try and contain all of that jiggle.

In these moments of attack, I acknowledge the voices and proceed to work toward my goals. The best thing about that voice is that it's just a voice. The power of life and death lies in the tongue, not in the mind.

Speak victory in these times of attack. There were moments when I would hear this voice then, take it captive, and then complete a run.

I wanted to scream and beat my chest in the end because I demolished the thought. This is a battle that you, too, can win. This is monumental, especially when you're unclear and can't decipher an ordained path due to the emotional and environmental fog. I'm a major advocate of mental health and spiritual centeredness. Our spirituality and awareness serve as an anchor to our mission, and our mission serves as the anchor to drive.

The Lifestyle Plan

If you're struggling to get to the gym, I'm almost certain your organization skills are subpar and more than likely nonexistent. Our normal day-to-day is hard to keep up with life if you're a serial entrepreneur and mother or father of multiple children. It's practically impossible. It's challenging to commit to researching and purchasing healthy food. If you're anything like me, you would have cleaned the kitchen and fridge, making room for beautifully prepped meals that would not make it out of the fridge because you forgot to pack them for work the next day, and now your food has expired.

If you have the time, great! Have at it. But if you don't, here's what I suggest:

Think about what you want to eat and where you will get it from. Finding healthy food on the go is often difficult if you do not plan ahead. Why is healthy food so inaccessible? It's the least convenient to find when you're on the go. I can't tell you how often I've been on family outings and vacations, and everyone's filling up on fast food. If I'm not equipped with my armor of snacks, I will fall victim to the trans-fat trap.

Armor yourself with snacks! Just as a soldier is always armed with a weapon in battle. In the car, in your purse, at work, or on your desk, snacks and water are protection from relapsing back to the unhealthy addicted eating habits you've kicked. I'm always equipped with a banana, an apple, nuts (peanuts, cashews, or almonds), and bottled water. Let's take a look at the food essentials I arm myself with. Better yet, let's look at my full grocery list.

Here's my grocery list:

Coffee
Bananas
Oat Milk
Peanut Butter
Vegan Protein (your choice)
Frozen Strawberries
Blueberries
Ginger Root
Spinach or Spring mix
Eggs
Avocados
Agave
Tomatoes
Nuts (Almonds, Cashews)
Ezekiel Bread
PAM
Salmon
Frozen Mixed Veggies
Bottled Water
Stevia
Apples

If you're allergic to any of these recommendations, you can substitute them with anything containing similar macronutrients. Also, if you eat meat, I recommend adding lean protein to your list.

No Matter what you do, if you follow these tips, the weight will fall off!

1. Eat within 12-hour windows. For example, I eat from 8 am-8 pm.
2. Drink half of your weight of water each day. I'm 123lbs, meaning I need to drink at least 62 ounces of water daily. Always round up!
3. Cut starch, sodas, and non-complex carbs.
4. Use Stevia instead of sugar (natural sweeteners like honey, agave, and maple syrup are also great alternatives.
5. No alcohol.
6. Minimize dairy. Use milk alternatives like almond, cashew, or oat milk.
7. Load up on the snacks (fruit, veggies, and nuts).
8. Repeat!

Variety is overrated!

Major Hack Alert: I eat the same thing every day. When something works for me, I allow it to keep working. That's also another way to ensure your success! Know what works for you.

Switching it up is okay once you find a system that works, but I highly recommend keeping it simple for the first 30 days. In doing this, you can lose up to 15 pounds in one month.

A Walk Through My Routine

When I awake in the morning, the first thing I do is fill up on water. I feel like it helps me get off to a healthy start. Not to mention if you need a water intake hack, the earlier you start, the better. If you start drinking water at 8 a.m., you can reach your goal by 4 p.m. if you drink one 16.9 oz bottle every two hours. Remember, strive to drink at least half of your body weight.

Here's what I eat in a day:
(If you are not pescatarian you can substitute all meat with a lean protein of your preference)

16.9 oz of bottled water

Morning snack:
Coffee or Tea and Apple

Breakfast option:
Garden Omelet with fruit or a 12 oz. smoothie (banana, peanut butter, spinach, protein, strawberries, blueberries, oat milk, and ginger)

16.9 oz of bottled water

Snack:
Almonds or Cashews

16.9 oz of bottled water

Lunch option:
Salad with grilled shrimp and low sugar vinegar-based dressings

16.9 oz of bottled water

Dinner option:
Grilled salmon (lean protein), 1 cup of quinoa (if you don't eat quinoa you can substitute for sweet potatoes, brown rice, or another complex carb), and mixed vegetables

16.9 oz of bottled water

Dinner and lunch options are interchangeable

This is typically where I end my evening. However, if you're still hungry, go ahead and have another snack.

Evening Snack Options:
Nut butters and veggies
Fruit
Avocado slices
Hummus
Smoothie

Plan, Plan, Plan

I encourage you to plan your meals. Meal planning is so much easier than meal prepping. Meal planning is my secret weapon. For example, if I know what I want to eat for lunch when I'm having breakfast, I have it delivered to me by lunchtime if I cannot make it.

Keep in mind that it is very much about progress, not perfection. If you slip up (I don't mean like slip up and eat a cheeseburger), I mean slip up and put ranch on your salad instead of a balsamic vinaigrette, don't allow slip-ups to cost you more than 200 calories. Between you and I, we can hardly afford that much.

Notice that I didn't put very much emphasis on what you can't have. We're not worried about that. Your body will adjust to your new routine!

If you end up eating dinner a little later than planned, that's okay. My only recommendation is that you eat no more than 2 hours before you go to bed. This is to allow your body time to metabolize what you ate.

Success Methods

I highly recommend downloading a calorie counting app for guidance. In case you detour from this regimen, the app will help you improvise. Search the food and find the macronutrient content before indulging. Utilizing this meal planning tactic will make you more likely to succeed.

Limit your environments and social activities for the first week so you can get adjusted. Get yourself accustomed to this new way of life.

Portion control is also a major key to your success. When I have something big for dinner or lunch, I split it in half. We don't need to eat it all in one sitting. We're no longer the child sitting at the dinner table with our parents or grandparents telling us that we'd better eat all of our food or, as my family would say, "clean that plate."

Eating more small meals throughout the day helps your metabolism stay high, which means you'll be burning fat faster. The longer you wait before eating, the more your body holds on to the food for survival because it doesn't know the next time it will be fed. It stores the food in your body instead of releasing it.

All in all, what worked best for me was a non-processed, plant-based, pescatarian diet and intermittent fasting. It's taken me a long time to share my weight loss journey recipe of success. I wasn't always confident, considering I am not a nutritionist or fitness expert. That's all the more reason why this may work for you. It's worked for me twice! I figured if it works for me, it can work for someone else. However, as I previously mentioned, I encourage you to consult with a professional and tailor this to your lifestyle as much as possible.

Water and Rest

As cliché as it may sound, resting is a major key to having a successful wellness experience. When you're sleep-deprived, your decisions are not well managed. Typically, you're functioning in the "whatever is convenient" capacity. You make better choices with a rested body. I find that I make impulsive eating choices when I have not had enough rest. It's ideal to get at least 8 hours of sleep. This is an attainable goal with an established routine.

Caffeine

Another dysfunctional relationship I've developed since the birth of my children is my relationship with coffee. When I discovered how alert and awake I felt after drinking coffee, I never turned back. It started with a caramel latte, just a single shot, then a single became a double, the double became triple, and then I hit a quad. I knew in that moment it was time to reel it in. My caffeine intake was getting out of control. Again, I'm not in the business of allowing a substance to control me. This dependency became something that I couldn't allow to get between me and my goals. Easier said, right?

It's not an easy habit to shake. I still drink it in moderation today—no more triple shots dressed in caramel and creams.

We always hear the cons about coffee, but here are some pros:

- It happens to reduce advancements of fibrosis and liver disease
- Your body processes sugar better; you're less likely to get type 2 diabetes.
- It's filled with antioxidants.
- It's correlated to a lower risk for diseases such as heart disease and Parkinson's.

My next major reason for drinking coffee was because it is an appetite suppressant. When I learned this, I looked to it for much more than just a wake-up call. I strategically had coffee each morning in preparation to subside my potential hunger before the start of my day. It would keep me awake and full. However, one with no health constraints should only consume 400mg of caffeine or less per day. Sometimes my intake exceeded that. Too much caffeine can result in seizures, abdominal pain, and an irregular heartbeat, which can be fatal, so it's important to keep it under control.

"*Purpose is priceless.*"

TAE RENÉ

19

Why Not, Wellness?

Wellness will instinctively become an intuitive habit each day. There are foods that I had to have every day that I no longer crave at all whatsoever. I will not name them because I do not want you to be triggered. There are also alternatives to your favorite foods that are just as fulfilling. Yes, there really are! Sometimes I would take the bread off a sandwich, wrap it with lettuce, pair it with an amazing salad, and be satisfied.

Keep your purpose before you. More important than knowing your why is to know your why not. I know exactly why I will not binge on ice cream and cookies at 10 pm. I channel that feeling of when I felt helpless and weak. This is actually an acting technique called substitution. Ask me how I know. That's for another book.

Knowing why not is more important than knowing why when it comes to weight loss and discipline because we are constantly learning and constantly evolving. Knowing your why not adds value to your worth. That makes all of the difference.

Yes, let's talk about that part. This is about reciprocating the value that we want the world to perceive. As a matter of fact, forget the world, forget other people, forget all of that. What about you? Don't you think you deserve to see the fruits of your wellness?

Don't you think you deserve the confidence you want to have when you step out into the world? This goes way beyond just feeling good about yourself or vanity metrics. This is so much bigger! Often when we don't recognize our value, we tolerate things in life that don't deserve us. That could be a dysfunctional relationship or even a career that underserves you and limits your growth.

If you're not living as your best self, accept accountability and change. Transitions in life are real and may come unexpectedly, causing you to discover mechanisms that help you cope. And it's okay. You might not be the best version of yourself today, but you can work toward it. The broken, exhausted, underappreciated, and overworked version of you deserves the time and space to develop into who you really are. Your body will follow your mind. Make the decision that your personal wellness matters and protect it from the old version of you. *I will plan my meals. I will eat healthy.* Decide and follow through.

Write down measurable sacrifices that you will make to achieve your goals:

_____

_____

_____

_____

_____

_____

_____

_____

Confidence hits differently when you carry out a plan that you created. The unforgiveness of others that you disguise in blame, the victimization, and all of the *could have, would have, should haves* end when showing up for yourself begins. Purpose is always the answer.

Focus on your purpose during this time. I mean, go for it! I don't mean pack up your home and move across the country but take the real estate class, take the headshots, apply for the job, complete the home project, initiate the relationship. Take the necessary steps to ultimately fulfilling your purpose. You deserve all of this and so much more.

"But when you find something worth suffering for, you're going to become someone you never thought you could be."
—Sarah Jakes Roberts

People's desires often supersede their work ethic. I would allow my daily routines to become distractions from my long-term goal. I avoided foreign concepts of discomfort and inconvenience. Of course, going to a fast-food restaurant and ordering your favorite combo is convenient, but if you want better for yourself, why continue to sabotage your future?

Think of it this way: you can feed what fuels your ambition or feed what fuels your complacency. That is the essence of transformative growth and meeting the best version of self. The wealth of the mind and willingness of self-discipline allows us to grow in spirit and truth.

Our greatest pursuit of wellness results in more than weight loss. This is a process of becoming by way of mental health, intentionality, and the pursuit of purpose. You may have realized that the entire book has about 10% of content directed toward diet plans and workouts. However, the physical work is a very small percentage of the battle. Your mental aptitude, spiritual temperament, and awareness are far more critical. Once I mastered the latter, I achieved far more than shedding pounds. I shed habits, toxic behaviors, and fears that revealed my faith beyond measure.

My 3-Day Theory

In scripture, several implications confirm the theory that there is significant meaning in a 3-day course. There are 27 occurrences in the Bible that transpired in 3 days. Three days is referenced 75 times in the Holy script. For brevity, we won't acknowledge each occurrence.

- Joseph releases his brother from prison in Egypt. (Genesis 42:17)
- On the third day, King Hezekiah is healed of an incurable disease. (2 Kings 20:5)
- The Israelites cross the Jordan River and take possession of the land as God's gift. (Joshua 1:11)
- "We must go a three days journey into the wilderness and sacrifice to the Lord our God as he commands us" (Exodus 8:27).

And the two most significant incidents.

- On the third day, the earth brought forth vegetation: seed-bearing plants of every kind and trees bearing fruit. (Genesis 1:12)
- The biggest highlight of them all is Jesus' resurrection. (I Corinthians 15:4)

It might appear an allegorical coincidence to some, but if an occurrence of death transcends to life in a matter of 3 days for Jesus, imagine then the demise of our old habits made anew in 3 days. As my mother says, *"Give it three days..."* My mother has always been a woman of great wisdom, but this guidance was prolific.

In parallel, it takes three days to break a habit. We're not talking about addiction. We're talking about habits. A habit is the tendency to do things without thinking, while addiction is doing something with no ability to stop even though it causes harm to you and potentially others.

On day one, you'll experience withdrawals each time you face temptation, attempting not to allow your cravings to overtake you. *Why am I putting myself through this? You'll frequently ask yourself, when can I indulge my cravings and free myself from this unnecessary pressure? I don't need to take on any more stress. I'm already overwhelmed with life's demands.*

In the earlier phases, it will feel like self-inflicted pain. You'll contemplate the value if this cycle of withdrawal persists. You surely wouldn't willingly put yourself through this daily. At the waking of day two, you'll be in disbelief at how you survived day one, yes! In excitement, you'll undress and run to your scale only for it not to reflect your efforts.

What seemed like it should produce instantaneous results will be a product of long-term discipline. On day three, you'll awake and cry. *Must I do this again?* In grievance, you'll muster the courage to follow through. You've lost two pounds. What will it hurt? The survival of day three is when the light gleams through the jagged cracks of defeat, and you'll be overwhelmed with hope. It's day four, and you're ready to take on the world.

Commit to one day at a time. Days become weeks, weeks become months, and you've lost ten pounds before you know it. Ten becomes 20, and you're coasting in your new life and body.

*P*ostpartum Awareness

I can now identify a victim of postpartum depression from a mile away, but unfortunately, there have been cases too close for comfort. A beautiful woman that worked her entire life for all of the scholarly accolades was passionate about her future, graduated from medical school, married a well-established guy, had two beautiful children, and you would presume lived happily ever after. She abandoned her husband just shy of 2 years into the marriage. Why? She had the perfect life from the outside looking in.

As I reflect on the years of servicing her as a client, I witnessed her working hard for the approval of peers and putting her truth on the backburner. Living for the validation of others became underwhelming.

She achieved every dream and goal she set, which contributed to the picture-perfect version of herself. After her accomplishments, she realized living her life based on other people's approval resulted in no longer appreciating or recognizing herself.

Can you imagine? You've devoted your entire life to something only to learn that it's not something you want? You look in the eyes of the children you've birthed to affirm that very thought, only for it to distance you further from your truth. Then you feel guilty for not wanting the lifestyle you chose because the desire never sets in. Your internal levee breaks and springs you into the life of a woman that you don't recognize. She ran with her children, and they lived in her car. She had to lose everything so that she could find herself.

When a mutual associate contacted me with this news, I said to myself, "Wow." I understood exactly what she was going through. At this time, I was in the process of renovating my own life. Often we don't give ourselves the time or separation necessary to learn our needs because it's not accommodated — falling victim to our emotions and fears, allowing them to overtake us. The mind is our greatest battlefield.

"As a man thinketh so is he."
—Proverbs 23:7, KJV

If you take a moment to dissect the verse of Solomon in Proverbs 23, start on the outside. Look at the verse from its exterior to diagnose the interior. This verse is better understood if you begin with the outcome and route it to the origin. If a man thinks and never acts, his life will reflect what he thinks regardless. No matter what, whether it manifests greatly or destructively. What you believe about yourself will be reflected in some area of your life or another.

It all stems from the inside. How you relate to yourself emotionally and spiritually is seen daily through your actions. Unhealthy eating habits begin with beautifully foiled, faultless excuses that have not been unwrapped with true knowledge of wellness. As a man thinketh, so is he, and so are you.

As a man thinketh, so is he, and so are you.

"The only way out is through."
—Tae René

Emotionally I began to deal. I started confronting my feelings face-on—even the uncomfortable ones. I'd been masking my fears in lies for so long that my issues were buried so deep that it would take an excavator to dig them up. Those layers served as protection for me. All of those suppressed emotions and feelings undealt resulted in emotional eating and drinking. The only way out is through. Fears, vulnerability, trauma, and disappointment are hard realities. Deal with that head-on. You're ready.

There were many things over the years that I had never confronted about my pain. I learned that the weight wasn't mine to carry; however, it manifested in other ways because I internalized my anger. Sometimes what looks like our barest effort is our greatest. The discipline that you exercise on a daily basis often goes unnoticed. For example, though you would have felt warranted in flying off the handle when insulted by the bank teller or local grocer, you activated our inner Michelle Obama – going high when they went low. This ability is a superpower that we will consistently practice throughout our wellness journey, it's called self-control.

Greatness is accessible to you. You have to decide exactly what you want in life and how you want to show up for it. Even if that means you simply want to improve as a person. Mastering the art of celebrating your wins without applause can only strengthen your spiritual endurance.

Think of your weight as an investment. Weight loss is the biggest return on investment that you can get. If calories are an expense and you have an allotted budget of 1500 calories for the day (for example), you're not going to waste it all in one place. You will manage this allowance wisely in an effort not to overspend.

"Her emotional wardrobe
of strength and dignity
will be inherited for
generations to come."

TAE RENÉ

20

Heirs of Strength

Learning should begin at home. Early on, I made it my mission to introduce a foundation of healthy habits to my girls. My oldest often struggled with consistency in eating healthy. I figured, what better lifestyle change to introduce her to than the MGC diet? I told her all about it, and she eagerly took on the task of Making Good Choices. She was excited and doing so well for the first few weeks, until one night it changed.

I was helping her get ready for bed. I always pick her clothes out for each school eve of the week. I laid out some cute skinny jeans with a pink sequin-embroidered top for a dress-down day.

"Mommy, can I wear tights to school tomorrow?" she asked.

Like most mothers, I have reservations about her attire because she is a beautifully developing young girl. I ensure that it's age-appropriate and is not exposing her prematurely. However, I almost instinctively knew that this fashion selection was the root of something much deeper.

Fully aware, I questioned, "What's been up with you and these tights lately, baby?"

Her eyes and mine locked briefly.

"Is it because your jeans aren't fitting you?"

Covered in pre-adolescent tears, her glassy eyes gazed upon my raised eyebrows and tilted head of honey blonde curls as I sat across from her.

"Are you strong?" I asked her.

In self-pity, she looked at me perplexed. "Yes, but I keep trying to eat healthy, and I can't," she confessed in fear of disappointing me, unsure if her tears disqualified her from my honor.

My laughter took her by surprise.

"What's so funny?" she asked.

"Who's in control of what you eat?"

"Me," she sighed.

"Do you remember seeing mommy run on the track when I was bigger?"

"Yes."

"That was very challenging. Do you see how making good choices worked for me? You got this! Don't cry about the things that you can control. You understand?" I said with my finger pointed and lips tight.

It was a gesture reminiscent of the exact way my mom pursed her lips when she meant what she said, leaving no room to inaccurately discern the gravity of her words.

"Yes, ma'am," she replied with her chin up militantly.

Deep down, she hoped that she could deliver on this abrupt initiation.

Granting her a little more strategy, I continued, "Give it three days, and it will get easier for you, I promise."

"Okay," she smiled as we embraced.

She went to her closet and grabbed more than a substitute wardrobe piece. This was the birth of her emotional wardrobe collection. Three weeks after our conversation, my oldest went to school in those jeans buttoned comfortably because she decided to show up for herself.

I wholeheartedly believe you now have the capacity to overcome postpartum, lose the physical and emotional weight, and keep it off for good. Not only did my daughter and I show up for ourselves we are living proof if you transform your mind; you will transform your life. The impact of your metamorphosis ignites irrevocable courage, aligns you with purpose, and brings stability to your legacy for generations.

You deserve to S.U.T.Y.

Love,

Website: **Taerene.com**
Instagram: **@Taetv**

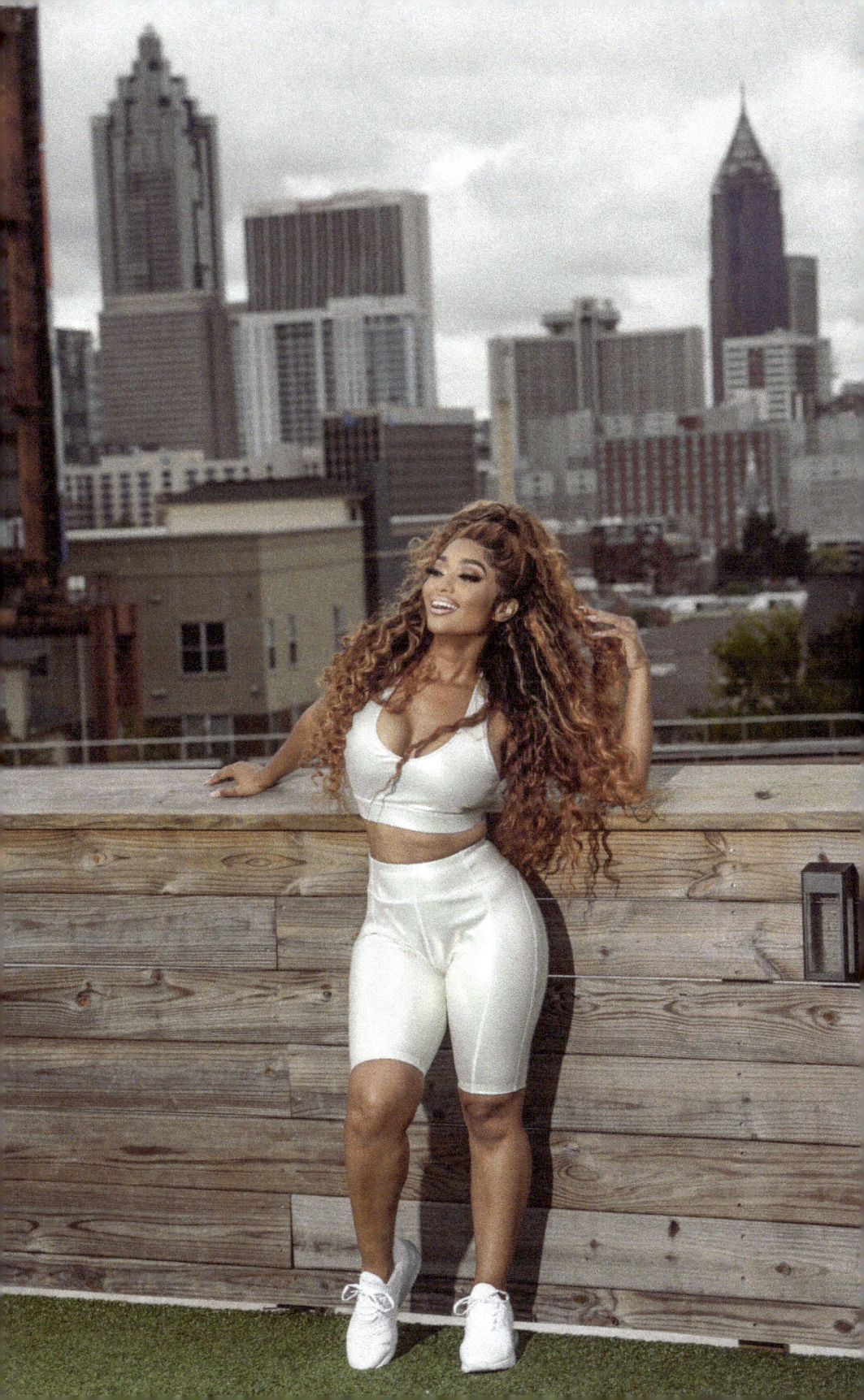

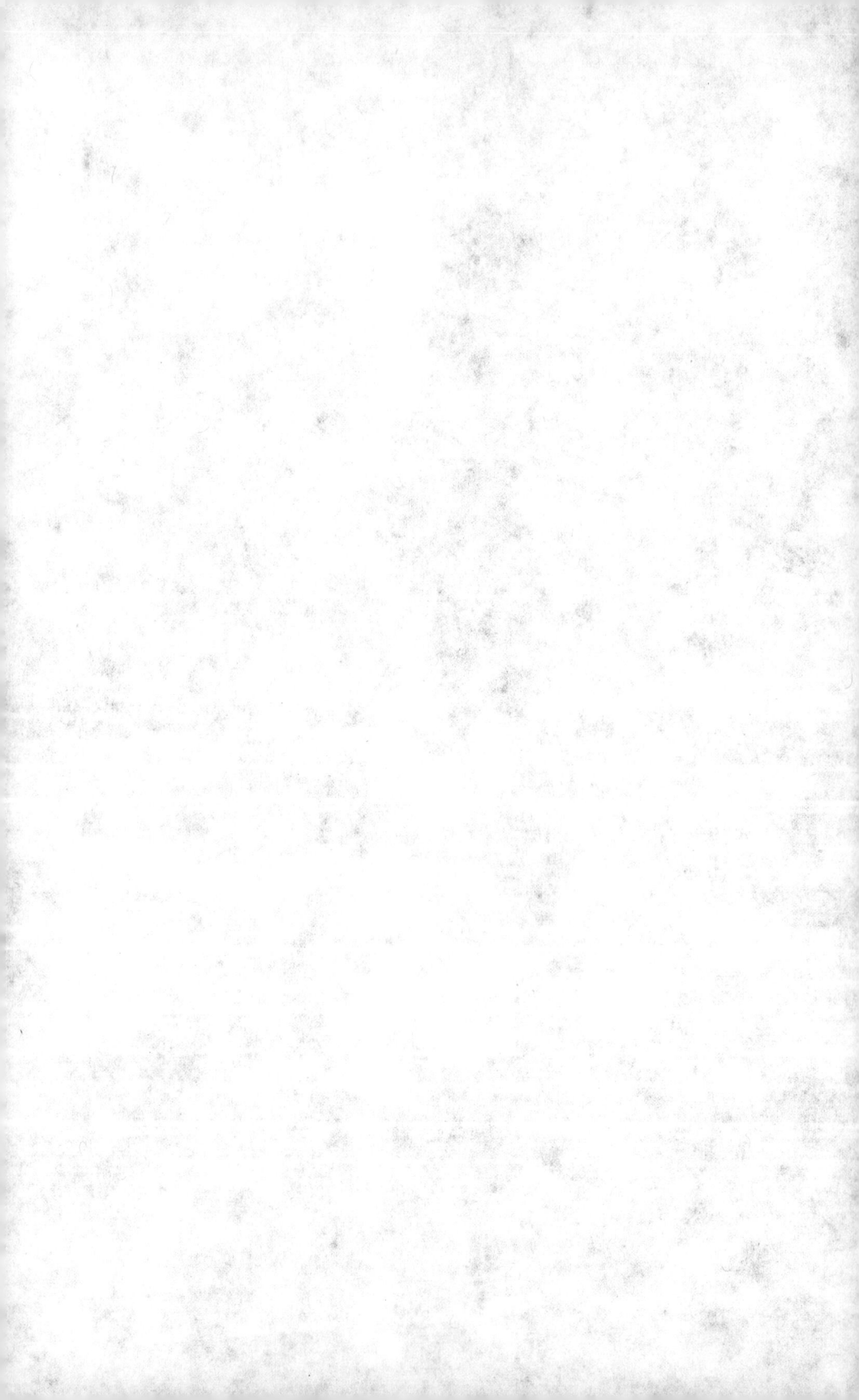